Knee Pain

Easy Exercises To Relieve And Prevent Knee Pain

(Best Knee Relief Exercises For Knee Pain, Arthritis, Stiffness, Rehabilitation)

Micheal Lee

I0089846

Published By **Darby Connor**

Micheal Lee

All Rights Reserved

*Knee Pain: Easy Exercises To Relieve And Prevent
Knee Pain (Best Knee Relief Exercises For Knee
Pain, Arthritis, Stiffness, Rehabilitation)*

ISBN   978-1-7772262-5-1

Legal & Disclaimer

The information contained in this book is not designed to replace or take the place of any form of medicine or professional medical advice. The information in this book has been provided for educational & entertainment purposes only.

The information contained in this book has been compiled from sources deemed reliable, and it is accurate to the best of the Author's knowledge; however, the Author cannot guarantee its accuracy and validity and cannot be held liable for any errors or omissions. Changes are periodically made to this book. You must consult your doctor or get professional medical advice before using any of the suggested remedies, techniques, or information in this book.

Table Of Contents

Chapter 1: Understanding Bad Knees

Common Causes of Knee Problems

Knee troubles are a common problem which can have an effect on people of every age and walks of life. These troubles can variety from moderate pain to immoderate ache and might significantly impact one's high-quality of life. Understanding the not unusual reasons of knee troubles is vital for prevention, early intervention, and powerful manipulate. In this text, we'll find out a number of the most common culprits inside the lower back of knee problems.

1.   Osteoarthritis: Osteoarthritis is one of the most important motives of knee pain, especially in older adults. This degenerative joint ailment takes area whilst the cartilage inside the knee joint wears down over the years, ensuing in pain, swelling, and decreased mobility.

2.   Injuries: Traumatic accidents, which consist of torn ligaments (just like the ACL,

MCL, or PCL) or meniscus tears, are a common reason of knee issues. These injuries often rise up in the path of sports activities activities sports activities or accidents and might result in massive ache and instability.

three. Overuse and Wear and Tear: Repetitive sports activities or overuse of the knee joint can result in situations like patellofemoral ache syndrome or tendinitis. These situations are characterized through ache throughout the kneecap or in the tendons that join the muscle mass to the knee.

4.   Obesity: Excess frame weight can placed extremely good strain on the knee joints, main to wear and tear, and increasing the chance of osteoarthritis. Maintaining a healthful weight is important for knee fitness.

five.   Rheumatoid   Arthritis: Rheumatoid arthritis is an autoimmune illness that may have an effect at the joints, collectively with the knees. It can purpose infection, pain, and swelling within the knee joint, most important to joint damage over time.

6.   Gout: Gout is a shape of arthritis due to the buildup of uric acid crystals inside the joints, in conjunction with the knees. It can result in sudden and immoderate ache, frequently referred to as "gout assaults."

7.   Bursitis: Knee bursitis takes vicinity on the same time as the bursae (small sacs packed with fluid) across the knee come to be inflamed because of overuse or trauma. This can motive ache, swelling, and confined mobility.

8.   Infections: Infections in or across the knee joint are significantly unusual however can purpose crucial knee problems if left untreated. Symptoms may also embody ache, swelling, redness, and fever.

nine. Genetics: Some humans can be predisposed to knee problems due to genetic elements. Conditions like familial osteoarthritis can boom the danger of growing knee problems.

10.   Age: As we age, the chance of developing knee problems honestly will increase. The put on and tear on the knee joints over the years can bring about conditions like osteoarthritis.

Prevention and control techniques for knee issues frequently encompass maintaining a healthy weight, everyday exercise to strengthen the muscle groups throughout the knee joint, the usage of proper techniques during bodily sports activities, and looking for spark off scientific hobby if injuries or symptoms and signs and symptoms upward push up. If you revel in persistent knee pain or soreness, it's vital to visit a healthcare professional for a proper prognosis and personalized treatment plan. Early intervention can assist alleviate signs and symptoms and signs and signs and enhance the prolonged-term health of your knees.

Diagnosing Your Specific Knee Issues

Knee pain and discomfort may be a demanding and debilitating experience.

Whether you're an athlete managing a sports activities-associated harm or an individual experiencing chronic knee pain, understanding the manner of diagnosing your unique knee troubles is crucial to finding effective treatment and comfort. In this article, we'll discover the steps involved in identifying and diagnosing knee problems.

1.   Medical History: The journey to a analysis regularly starts offevolved offevolved with a speak of your medical facts. Your healthcare enterprise will ask about your symptoms, when they started out, and any past injuries or situations that can be associated with your knee pain. This data allows offer context for the evaluation.

2.   Physical Examination: A thorough bodily examination is vital for assessing your knee's range of motion, balance, and commonplace circumstance. Your healthcare issuer will search for signs and symptoms of swelling, tenderness, or deformity and can

carry out particular assessments to evaluate ligament and muscle characteristic.

3.   Imaging Studies: To get a more unique view of the knee joint and surrounding structures, imaging studies may be advocated. Common imaging equipment embody X-rays, that might display bone problems like fractures or arthritis, and MRI (Magnetic Resonance Imaging), which gives a clean picture of mild tissues together with ligaments and cartilage.

four. Laboratory Tests: In a few instances, blood checks may be essential to rule out underlying conditions like rheumatoid arthritis or gout, that can affect the knee joint.

5.   Diagnostic Injections: In instances wherein the supply of knee ache is uncertain, a diagnostic injection can be administered. This includes injecting a neighborhood anesthetic or anti-inflammatory remedy into the knee joint to determine if it alleviates the

ache. If the ache subsides quickly, it may assist pinpoint the deliver of the hassle.

6.   Specialized Tests: Depending on the suspected difficulty, your healthcare enterprise can also moreover recommend specialized assessments. For example, an arthroscopy is a minimally invasive way wherein a small virtual digital digicam is inserted into the knee joint to straight away visualize the internal structures and make a assessment.

7.   Consulting with Specialists: Depending at the complexity of your knee hassle, your number one care medical doctor may additionally moreover moreover refer you to a representative, collectively with an orthopedic fitness care organisation or a rheumatologist, for a higher evaluation.

Once your precise knee problem is identified, your healthcare agency will talk remedy options with you. Treatment plans variety appreciably depending at the diagnosis however may additionally encompass physical remedy, medicine, injections, way of life adjustments, or, in a few instances, surgery.

It's vital to be proactive in searching for a diagnosis for knee ache or pain. Ignoring or neglecting knee troubles can purpose worsening conditions, reduced mobility, and a discounted high-quality of lifestyles. Additionally, early analysis and treatment frequently result in extra a fulfillment results and a faster move returned to an active and pain-free manner of lifestyles.

Remember that everyone's knee troubles are particular, and the diagnostic manner may additionally differ for this reason. Always go to a licensed healthcare agency to make sure an correct evaluation and to accumulate the most suitable and powerful remedy in your specific knee problems.

The Impact of Bad Knees on Mobility

Mobility is a vital component of our every day lives, permitting us to transport, carry out duties, and revel in sports activities independently. However, when horrible knees come into the photograph, mobility can be substantially compromised. Knee problems, whether or no longer because of damage, arthritis, or other factors, have a profound effect on an person's functionality to transport freely and effortlessly. In this article, we'll discover the various methods awful knees have an effect on mobility and communicate capability answers.

1.   Pain and Discomfort: The maximum on the spot and vital effect of terrible knees on mobility is pain. Knee pain can variety from moderate ache to intense, throbbing suffering, making even the most effective movements a undertaking. Individuals with terrible knees frequently revel in pain at the same time as walking, status, or perhaps sitting for extended periods.

2.   Stiffness: Bad knees can bring about stiffness in the joint, making it difficult to bend or straighten the knee completely. This can limit activities like mountain climbing

stairs, getting into and out of chairs, and kneeling.

3.   Reduced Range of Motion: The flexibility and kind of motion inside the knee joint can be significantly restrained with the aid of conditions like osteoarthritis or injuries. This impediment impacts the capability to participate in sports that require bending, squatting, or twisting motions.

four. Instability: Instability is a common trouble with horrible knees. Individuals may additionally experience as despite the fact that their knees are wobbly or about to offer way, growing the risk of falls. This fear of instability can in addition restriction mobility as individuals become extra careful in their actions.

five. Difficulty with Weight-Bearing Activities: Activities that contain bearing weight on the knees, together with strolling or recognition for prolonged periods, grow to be mainly hard for those with knee issues.

The ache and pain can lead to a sedentary way of life.

6.   Impact on Everyday Tasks: Everyday obligations like getting dressed, bathing, and cooking can also end up exhausting for human beings with horrific knees. Simple actions like stepping into a bath or stepping into and out of a vehicle can become essential stressful conditions.

7.   Reduced Independence: The loss of mobility because of lousy knees can reason decreased independence. Individuals may additionally furthermore want help with daily obligations, and they'll avoid going out or socializing due to the restrictions imposed with the aid of manner in their knees.

eight. Emotional Impact: The frustration and emotional toll of residing with lousy knees need to no longer be underestimated. Individuals may additionally moreover moreover revel in feelings of helplessness, melancholy, or anxiety, in particular if their knee problems are persistent and extended-lasting.

Addressing the impact of awful knees on mobility frequently includes a multi-faceted method

Consultation with Healthcare Professionals: Seeking clinical advice and remedy options is important. Healthcare companies can provide diagnoses, prescribe appropriate medicines, and endorse physical remedy.

Physical Therapy: Physical therapists can growth tailor-made exercise packages to decorate knee strength, flexibility, and mobility.

Assistive Devices: Mobility aids inclusive of canes, crutches, or knee braces can offer assist and stability.

Chapter 2: Setting the Right Mindset

The Psychological Aspect of Staying Active After 60

As we age, staying lively becomes no longer handiest a physical necessity but furthermore a vital detail in keeping our mental nicely-being. While the physical advantages of exercise are properly-documented, the effect on highbrow health and common happiness can not be overstated. In this newsletter, we find out the profound highbrow issue of staying lively after 60.

1. Mood Elevation: Regular bodily interest triggers the discharge of endorphins, the body's natural temper lifters. These "enjoy-correct" chemical compounds assist fight feelings of disappointment, tension, and depression. Staying active can appreciably decorate your preferred mood and emotional properly-being.

2. Stress Reduction: Life can be demanding at any age, however as we come to be older, we can also stumble upon extra

stressors associated with health, budget, or family. Engaging in bodily hobby is an effective way to govern and reduce strain tiers. Exercise presents an opportunity to step a long way from each day concerns and popularity at the prevailing moment.

three. Enhanced Cognitive Function: Staying energetic has been related to superior cognitive characteristic and a reduced hazard of cognitive decline. Exercise stimulates the mind, enhances memory, and sharpens cognitive skills, assisting older adults stay mentally agile.

four. Boosted Self-Esteem: The enjoy of fulfillment that comes with achieving health desires can improve self-esteem and self-self belief. This is specifically crucial as vanity can every so often take successful with age-related modifications in appearance or physical skills.

five. Social Connection: Participating in group sports or exercising education gives an possibility for social interaction and constructing connections. Social engagement is vital for keeping intellectual and emotional health, and staying energetic may be a a laugh and social manner to fulfill new human beings and improve current relationships.

6. Sense of Purpose: Many older adults discover that staying lively offers them a experience of motive and course. Whether it's pursuing a ultra-modern-day fitness intention, participating in community activities, or volunteering, physical activity can add because of this that and achievement to lifestyles.

7. Better Sleep: Regular bodily interest can improve the high-quality of sleep. Restful sleep is important for emotional resilience, attention, and ordinary intellectual well-being.

8. Reduction of Isolation: As people age, they may face stepped forward isolation, that could lead to emotions of loneliness and melancholy. Staying lively can provide a motive to go away the residence, interact

with others, and combat the terrible results of isolation.

9. Positive Outlook on Aging: Maintaining an active way of existence can help older adults encompass ageing with a outstanding outlook. It annoying conditions stereotypes about what it way to grow old, demonstrating that lifestyles can live colourful and pleasant properly into the senior years.

10. Stress Coping Mechanism: Facing the demanding situations that regularly encompass growing older, together with fitness troubles or loss of loved ones, may be emotionally taxing. Staying energetic can feature a healthful coping mechanism, helping people navigate these lifestyles changes more efficiently.

In summary, the mental benefits of staying energetic after 60 are severa and profound. Regular bodily interest can result in stepped forward temper, reduced stress, greater relevant cognitive feature, expanded conceitedness, and a greater enjoy of purpose. It's now not quite plenty staying match; it's approximately dwelling a happier, more exciting life in the later years. So, lace up those footwear, encompass an active life-style, and delight inside the top notch impact it is able to have for your intellectual and emotional well-being.

Overcoming Fears and Doubts

Embarking on an active way of existence adventure after the age of 60 can be a daunting prospect for plenty. Fears and doubts often creep in, making it seem like an uphill battle. However, with the right mind-set and method, you can conquer those limitations and include the benefits of staying energetic for your golden years. In this article, we'll find out a few common fears and doubts associated with staying energetic after 60 and provide guidance on conquering them.

1.   Fear of Injury: One of the maximum huge concerns is the priority of having injured finally of bodily hobby. After 60, the body might not get better as speedy because it as

quickly as did. However, the key is to start slowly and select low-impact activities that reduce the hazard of damage. Gentle sporting sports like taking walks, swimming, or yoga may be exquisite starting factors.

2.   Doubt About Physical Abilities: Doubts approximately your bodily capabilities also can maintain you again from staying lively. It's important to understand that you don't need to be a health guru to enjoy the benefits of workout. Everyone starts offevolved offevolved someplace, and even small efforts may additionally need to make a large difference to your fitness and fitness.

three. Lack of Motivation: Maintaining motivation may be hard at any age, however it can feel even greater daunting as you turn out to be old. To combat this, set easy and attainable goals, and find out an exercise ordinary which you sincerely experience. Consider exercise with a friend or becoming a member of a health splendor for brought motivation and duty.

four.   Feeling Self-Conscious: Some humans can also sense self-aware about their look or health diploma at the same time as beginning an energetic manner of existence later in life. Remember that you're doing this for your self and your health, not to affect others. Focus on your journey and development as opposed to comparing yourself to others.

5.   Chronic Health Conditions: If you have persistent fitness situations, you may in all likelihood worry that exercise want to exacerbate them. However, many fitness conditions may be controlled and stepped forward through bodily interest. Consult at the side of your healthcare company to develop a safe and tailor-made exercising plan that takes your particular health needs into attention.

6.   Time Constraints: A commonplace doubt is whether or now not or not you have got got enough time to your time table for regular workout. Prioritizing bodily hobby is critical to your health, and it's feasible to find

small pockets of time in some unspecified time within the destiny of the day for brief bouts of exercising. Incorporate bodily hobby into your ordinary gradually until it turns into a dependancy.

7.   Aging-Related Changes: It's natural for the frame to undergo modifications with age, which includes decreased muscles or joint stiffness. Instead of seeing those modifications as obstacles, view them as reasons to live active. Exercise can assist counteract the consequences of getting older and enhance your normal first-rate of lifestyles.

8.   Lack of Knowledge: If you're sudden with exercise sports activities and strategies, you may probably fear doing a little element wrong. Consider operating with a licensed fitness instructor or bodily therapist who can guide you very well and successfully.

Chapter 3: Low-Impact Exercise Options

Introduction to Low-Impact Exercises

Exercise is a critical thing of a healthy way of life, but it's not constantly approximately immoderate-intensity physical sports or strenuous sports activities. For people who need a gentler approach because of factors like joint troubles, accidents, or actually a desire for low-impact motion, there are hundreds of options available. In this article, we'll discover the area of low-effect physical games and their severa advantages.

What Are Low-Impact Exercises?

Low-impact carrying sports activities are physical sports activities that vicinity minimum strain at the joints and the body as a whole. These bodily video games offer a gentler manner to live active, making them suitable for human beings of all health stages, a while, and physical conditions. They are especially treasured for the ones convalescing from injuries, dealing with continual situations, or searching for to ease into an exercise ordinary.

Benefits of Low-Impact Exercises:

1.   Joint-Friendly: The primary gain of low-impact bodily games is their mild nature, which reduces the hazard of joint accidents and minimizes located on and tear on the frame.

2.   Accessible: Low-effect sports are available to almost anyone, regardless of age, fitness degree, or bodily limitations.

3.   Pain Management: For those managing continual ache or getting better from injuries, those physical activities can offer ache consolation and useful resource in rehabilitation.

4.   Cardiovascular Health: Many low-impact sports, together with swimming or cycling, offer incredible cardiovascular advantages without the jarring effect of excessive-impact workout exercises.

5.   Weight   Management: Low-effect sporting activities may be effective for coping with weight and promoting standard fitness with out straining the joints.

6.   Improved Balance and Coordination: Many low-effect activities involve balance and coordination, assisting individuals keep and decorate those essential abilities.

7.   Stress Reduction: Exercise, even in a low-impact form, triggers the discharge of endorphins, reducing strain and enhancing highbrow nicely-being.

Types of Low-Impact Exercises:

1.   Walking: One of the handiest however handiest low-effect bodily video games, strolling gives cardiovascular blessings and can be tailored to various health tiers.

2.   Swimming: Swimming is an brilliant entire-body exercise that is easy on the joints. It builds electricity, patience, and flexibility.

three. Cycling: Riding a motorcycle, whether or not outdoors or on a table positive motorbike, offers a low-impact way to enhance cardiovascular health and leg electricity.

4. Yoga: Yoga combines mild actions, stretches, and deep respiration to enhance flexibility, stability, and intellectual readability.

five. Tai Chi: Tai Chi is a sluggish and smooth martial art work that focuses on stability, flexibility, and rest. It's perfect for boosting posture and decreasing pressure.

6. Elliptical Trainer: This device offers a low-impact, entire-body exercise, making it an high-quality desire for individuals looking for to beautify cardiovascular fitness.

7. Pilates: Pilates specializes in middle electricity, flexibility, and trendy frame recognition. It can be tailored to splendid health stages and is known for its low-impact nature.

eight. Water Aerobics: Conducted in a pool, water aerobics gives resistance without the jarring effect of land-primarily based bodily sports. It's brilliant for joint guide and muscle firming.

In the following sections of this collection, we can delve deeper into each of those low-effect workout options, exploring their benefits, techniques, and tips for buying started out. Whether you're convalescing from an damage, handling a chronic circumstance, or in reality select out a mild method to health, low-effect bodily video video games offer a pathway to higher fitness and nicely-being. Stay tuned to discover which low-impact exercising might be the precise healthy for your life-style and health desires.

Benefits of Low-Impact Workouts: A Gentle Path to Health

Knee ache and pain may be enormous obstacles at the path to retaining an energetic and healthful way of life. Fortunately, low-impact sporting occasions offer a moderate but quite powerful way to stay in shape and shield your knees from in addition strain or harm. In this text, we'll find out the severa advantages of low-impact exercising workout routines, mainly for humans with awful knees.

1. Reduced Joint Stress:

One of the maximum sizeable blessings of low-impact exercising workouts is their capability to reduce stress at the knees and precise weight-bearing joints. Unlike excessive-effect bodily video games like strolling or jumping, low-effect sports consisting of swimming, biking, and strolling are gentler at the joints. This makes them an first-rate desire for people with awful knees who want to limit effect to relieve pain and save you in addition harm.

2. Pain Management:

Low-effect physical games can provide comfort from knee ache associated with situations like osteoarthritis or preceding accidents. The managed and fluid actions in wearing activities like yoga, tai chi, and water aerobics help growth joint flexibility, reduce stiffness, and alleviate pain, promoting normal knee health.

3. Joint Lubrication:

Regular low-effect sports can make contributions to higher joint lubrication. The repetitive, controlled motions concerned in sports like biking and elliptical training stimulate the manufacturing of synovial fluid, which lubricates the knee joint. This increased lubrication can enhance joint characteristic and decrease friction and pain.

4. Improved Muscle Strength:

Weak muscle tissues around the knee joint can contribute to knee problems and instability. Low-effect exercise workout routines, specifically folks who contain electricity schooling and resistance physical activities, assist construct muscle power with out straining the knees. Stronger leg muscle tissue offer higher manual for the knee joint, lowering the hazard of harm.

5. Cardiovascular Benefits:

Low-effect sports activities can deliver sizable cardiovascular blessings without placing undue stress on the knees. Activities like swimming and the usage of an elliptical system increase the heart rate and assist decorate cardiovascular fitness, fundamental to a greater in shape coronary heart and circulatory machine.

6. Weight Management:

Maintaining a healthy weight is vital for knee health. Excess body weight locations added pressure at the knees, exacerbating ache and soreness. Low-impact bodily video games may be part of a balanced approach to weight control, helping people shed extra kilos and alleviate stress on the knee joints.

7. Improved Balance and Flexibility:

Low-impact sports including yoga and tai chi awareness on stability, flexibility, and body popularity. These sports no longer most effective decorate knee stability however moreover decorate common frame coordination and posture, decreasing the risk of falls and injuries.

8. Long-Term Sustainability:

One of the critical issue benefits of low-impact workout routines is their lengthy-term sustainability. Unlike immoderate-effect physical video video games that would become much less possible as people age, low-impact activities continue to be on hand and interesting nicely into the senior years. This makes them an excellent desire for human beings seeking out a lifelong fitness solution.

In quit, low-impact exercise workouts offer a big type of benefits for human beings with lousy knees. By decreasing joint stress, handling ache, developing muscle strength, and assisting primary joint fitness, the ones slight physical video video games empower humans to maintain an energetic and healthy way of life at the same time as safeguarding their knees. Whether you're getting better from an injury, dealing with a chronic knee scenario, or really in search of a kinder method to health, low-impact sports may be your pathway to a ache-free and energetic existence.

Low effect precise workout sports

Exercise Routine for Bad Knees

Exercise is essential for preserving knee fitness and mobility, even when you have terrible knees. Here are some low-effect bodily games that can assist make stronger the muscle tissues spherical your knees and enhance ordinary joint stability. Remember to visit a healthcare employer or bodily therapist earlier than starting any new exercising software program application, specially if you have pre-current knee situations.

1. Leg Raises (Straight Leg Raises):

Lie flat on your decrease lower back with one leg bent and the other leg right now.

Tighten your thigh muscle corporations in the right away leg and raise it slowly, retaining it instantly, until it's parallel to the bent knee.

Hold for a few seconds, then lower your leg slowly.

Perform 2 gadgets of 10-15 reps for every leg.

2. Clamshells:

Lie to your facet on the facet of your knees bent at a ninety-degree angle and your ft together.

Keeping your ft touching, convey your pinnacle knee as immoderate as you without issue can on the identical time as retaining your balance.

Lower the knee backpedal.

Perform 2 units of 10-15 reps for each side.

3. Wall Sits:

Stand in conjunction with your yet again against a wall.

Slide down the wall till your knees are bent at a 90-degree attitude, as in case you were sitting in a chair.

Hold this role for as long as you can (start with 15-30 seconds and grade by grade increase the time).

Repeat 2-3 instances.

four. Seated Leg Raises:

Sit on a strong chair at the side of your ft flat at the floor.

Straighten one leg and lift it as immoderate as you effortlessly can.

Chapter 4: Strength and Flexibility Training

Building Strength and Flexibility: A Path to Pain Relief and Improved Mobility

Knee pain, whether or no longer due to arthritis, harm, or placed on and tear, may be a large barrier to an active and pain-loose existence. However, there's choice for those with horrible knees via strength and versatility education. In this newsletter, we'll find out how focused bodily games can assist alleviate pain, beautify knee function, and beautify ordinary first rate of life.

The Importance of Strength and Flexibility:

Before delving into particular bodily games, it's critical to apprehend the jobs that power and versatility play in managing knee pain:

1. Strength: Strong muscular tissues around the knee joint provide vital guide and balance. Strengthening physical games can help distribute the load greater gently and decrease stress on the knees.

2.   Flexibility: Maintaining or improving joint flexibility is similarly crucial. It allows make certain a complete form of movement, that might alleviate stiffness and pain.

Strength Training for Bad Knees:

1.   Leg Raises: Lie in your once more with one knee bent and the opportunity leg without delay. Tighten the thigh muscle mass of the right away leg and raise it slowly, maintaining it directly. Hold in quick, then lower it down. Repeat for every legs.

2.   Wall Sits: Stand at the facet of your lower back in the direction of a wall and slide down until your knees are bent at a 90-degree angle, as in case you're sitting in a chair. Hold this function for so long as you could, then return to a standing feature. This exercising strengthens the quadriceps.

3.   Seated Leg Press: Use a leg press tool on the health club or a resistance band at home. Sit down and press your legs outward,

straightening them in opposition to resistance.

four. Step-Ups: Stand within the the front of a step or sturdy platform. Step up with one leg after which step down. Repeat with the possibility leg. Use a railing or wall for assist if wished.

five. Bridges: Lie in your yet again with knees bent and toes flat at the floor. Lift your hips off the ground, keeping your toes and shoulders on the ground. This exercising engages the glutes and hamstrings.

Flexibility Exercises for Bad Knees:

1. Knee Flexor Stretch: Sit at the floor together collectively together with your legs directly. Bend one knee, bringing your heel inside the route of your buttocks. Gently maintain the pinnacle of your foot and pull it within the course of your buttocks to experience a stretch within the the front of the thigh. Hold for 20-30 seconds on each leg.

2.   Hamstring Stretch: Sit with one leg prolonged and the alternative bent so the only of your foot rests in the direction of your internal thigh. Lean in advance lightly to enjoy a stretch for your hamstring. Hold for 20-30 seconds and switch legs.

three. Quadriceps Stretch: Stand on one leg, defensive onto a wall or chair for stability. Bend your opposite knee, bringing your heel in the direction of your buttocks. Hold your ankle and lightly pull your foot in the direction of your buttocks to stretch the the front of your thigh. Hold for 20-30 seconds on each leg.

four.   Calf Stretch: Stand going through a wall at the side of your hands at the wall. Step one foot once more, maintaining it right now, and press the heel into the ground. Feel the stretch in your calf muscle. Hold for 20-30 seconds on every leg.

five.   IT Band Stretch: Stand with one foot crossed over the alternative. Lean to the component, feeling a stretch along the outer thigh. Hold for 20-30 seconds on every factor.

Remember to start with low resistance and brief durations, regularly growing as your knees grow to be more potent and extra flexible. Always talk with a healthcare company or physical therapist in advance than starting any exercising software for horrible knees, as they are capable of provide custom designed guidance and ensure that the sporting events are secure and appropriate on your specific scenario. With power of thoughts and consistency, power and flexibility training may be a sport-changer in coping with knee pain and enhancing your customary first-rate of life.

Building Strength to Support Your Knees: A Blueprint for Pain-Free Living

Knee pain can be a debilitating situation that limits your potential to transport freely and revel in lifestyles to the fullest. However, building energy in the muscular tissues surrounding your knees can be a effective approach for assuaging pain, enhancing joint balance, and regaining mobility. In this newsletter, we'll discover how you could make more potent key muscle businesses to beneficial aid your knees and embark on a direction to pain-free living.

Understanding the Importance of Muscle Strength for Knee Health:

The knees are one of the frame's number one weight-bearing joints. They undergo the burden of your frame and any extra weight you bring, making them prone to placed on and tear over time. When the muscle tissues throughout the knees are prone or imbalanced, the knee joint might also moreover enjoy prolonged strain, fundamental to pain, instability, and a better threat of harm.

Key Muscle Groups for Knee Support:

1.   Quadriceps: These muscle corporations at the the front of your thighs play a critical function in knee extension and balance. Weak

quadriceps can bring about joint instability and reduced wonder absorption.

2. Hamstrings: Located within the back of your thighs, the hamstrings art work in opposition to the quadriceps. Strengthening them allows hold knee joint stability and stability.

three. Glutes: The gluteal muscle tissues, specifically the gluteus medias and gluteus maximus, provide important assist to the hips and knees. Strong glutes help with proper alignment and reduce strain on the knees.

four. Calf Muscles: Strong calf muscle mass make a contribution to conventional decrease limb stability and can assist take in forces that could otherwise have an effect at the knee joint.

5. Hip Muscles: Muscles across the hips, which includes the hip abductors and adductors, play a position in retaining proper leg alignment. Strengthening these muscles can reduce knee strain.

Effective Exercises for Knee Support:

1.   Squats: Squats are a amazing compound exercising that goals the quadriceps, hamstrings, and glutes. Start with bodyweight squats and development to weighted squats as your power improves.

2.   Lunges: Walking lunges or desk certain lunges assist provide a boost to the quadriceps and hamstrings at the equal time as enhancing stability and coordination.

three. Leg Press: Leg press machines on the health club or resistance band leg presses at home can be effective for strengthening the quadriceps.

four. Deadlifts: Deadlifts are terrific for strengthening the hamstrings and glutes, however right form is critical to avoid harm. Consider operating with a trainer to make sure you're the use of correct method.

five.   Bridges: Lie on your yet again with knees bent and toes flat on the floor. Lift your hips off the ground to interact the glutes and hamstrings.

6. Step-Ups: Using a strong step or platform, step up with one leg after which step down. This workout lets in help the quadriceps and glutes.

7. Resistance Band Exercises: Utilize resistance bands for leg lifts, leg curls, and aspect leg will increase to aim precise muscle companies at some stage in the knees.

Safety Tips:

Start with low resistance and repetitions, regularly growing as your power improves.

Focus on proper form to avoid harm. Consider working with a certified fitness trainer or bodily therapist to take a look at correct method.

Listen on your body. If you experience ache or ache during an exercising, prevent and are looking for recommendation from a healthcare organisation.

By incorporating the ones physical video games into your fitness everyday and that specialize in strengthening the important thing muscle corporations that beneficial aid your knees, you could considerably reduce knee pain, decorate joint stability, and enjoy a more lively and pain-unfastened lifestyles. Remember that consistency is essential, and improvement may be sluggish, so be affected person and stay devoted on your electricity-building journey.

Improving Flexibility for Better Knee Joint Health: A Step Toward Pain-Free Living

Knee joint health is a critical component of not unusual properly-being, as our knees guide our every day moves and sports. One often overlooked but extraordinarily effective way to maintain wholesome knees is through improving flexibility. In this newsletter, we'll discover the importance of flexibleness for knee joint health and offer realistic suggestions that will help you obtain extra flexibility and decrease the risk of ache or harm.

Why Flexibility Matters for Knee Health:

1.   Enhanced Range of Motion: Flexibility sports assist improve the shape of motion to your knee joints. This way you can skip your knees thru their entire capability without discomfort or obstacles.

2.   Reduced Stiffness: Stiff knees can result in ache and ward off your capability to carry out normal sports activities. Stretching and versatility carrying sports activities help alleviate stiffness, making movement smoother and extra cushty.

three. Injury Prevention: Flexible muscle organizations and tendons are much less vulnerable to damage. By enhancing flexibility round your knees, you could reduce the chance of traces, sprains, and other knee-related injuries.

four. Pain Management: Flexibility carrying events can offer consolation from knee pain, specifically for humans with situations like osteoarthritis or continual knee discomfort. Gentle stretches can help ease anxiety and alleviate ache.

Effective Flexibility Exercises for Knee Joint Health:

1.   Quad Stretch: Stand up at once and produce your proper heel inside the route of your buttocks, keeping your ankle at the side of your proper hand. Gently pull your heel in the course of your buttocks to enjoy a stretch inside the front of your thigh. Hold for 20-30 seconds and repeat on the opposite leg.

2.   Hamstring Stretch: Sit collectively along with your legs extended within the front of you. Bend one knee, bringing the only of your foot in competition to the inner thigh of your opposite leg. Reach to your feet at the extended leg at the same time as preserving your lower decrease back proper away. Hold for 20-30 seconds and switch legs.

3.   Calf Stretch: Stand going via a wall and location your arms on it for assist. Step one foot again at the equal time as keeping it immediately, pressing your heel into the ground. Feel the stretch for your calf muscle. Hold for 20-30 seconds on every leg.

four.   IT Band Stretch: Stand on the side of your ft hip-width apart. Cross your proper leg at the back of your left and attain your right arm overhead, bending for your left aspect. You'll revel in a stretch along your outer thigh. Hold for 20-30 seconds and switch elements.

5.   Knee Flexor Stretch: Sit at the ground together together with your legs straight away. Bend one knee and convey your heel in the path of your buttocks. Hold the top of your foot together collectively together with your hand and lightly pull your foot toward your buttocks. Feel the stretch in the the the front of your thigh. Hold for 20-30 seconds on each leg.

6.   Butterfly Stretch: Sit with the soles of your toes collectively and your knees bent out

to the edges. Hold your toes together along side your arms and gently push your knees towards the floor to enjoy a stretch in your internal thighs and knees. Hold for 20-30 seconds.

Tips for Safe and Effective Stretching:

Warm up earlier than stretching with moderate cardio wearing sports like walking or biking to boom blood waft to your muscle tissue.

Stretch slowly and lightly, fending off any sharp or painful moves.

Hold each stretch for 20-30 seconds, breathing deeply and exciting into the stretch.

Perform stretches frequently, preferably as a part of your every day normal.

By incorporating the ones flexibility bodily games into your every day life, you can beautify knee joint fitness, reduce the threat of pain or harm, and enjoy extra freedom of motion. Remember that consistency is prime, and with time and persistence, you'll revel in the advantages of advanced knee flexibility and not unusual properly-being.

Guided Exercises and Routines Specifically for Stronger and Healthier Knees

Knee health is of paramount importance, as our knees play a pivotal characteristic in our mobility and every day sports. Whether you're seeking to relieve knee pain, get over an harm, or clearly need to hold your knees sturdy and flexible, guided bodily activities and exercises may be your remarkable allies. In this article, we'll discover the benefits of guided knee sports activities and offer a pattern regular that will help you in your journey to healthier knees.

Why Choose Guided Knee Exercises?

Guided knee bodily sports offer numerous benefits, in particular in case you're new to energy training or rehabilitation. Here's why they're a precious preference:

1.   Structured Approach: Guided exercises offer a based totally and systematic way to aim particular muscle companies at some stage in the knees.

2.   Expert Guidance: Many guided carrying occasions are designed and led via way of licensed health walking shoes or physical therapists, making sure that you purchased professional steering and education.

three. Safety: Guided physical video games often emphasize proper form and method, lowering the risk of harm or stress.

four. Variety: Guided wearing sports normally consist of loads of wearing events to engage exceptional muscle businesses, main to complete knee guide.

5.   Progress Tracking: Many guided workout applications provide development monitoring and feedback, allowing you to expose your improvement through the years.

Sample Guided Knee Exercise Routine:

Below is a easy guided knee exercising everyday to get you commenced out. Remember to are trying to find recommendation from a healthcare corporation or bodily therapist in advance than starting any new exercise software program, especially if you have pre-contemporary knee conditions.

1. Knee Flexor Stretch:

Start in a seated characteristic collectively at the side of your legs prolonged.

Bend one knee, bringing your heel toward your buttocks.

Hold the top of your foot in conjunction with your hand and lightly pull it towards your buttocks.

Feel the stretch inside the the front of your thigh.

Hold for 20-30 seconds and transfer legs.

2. Quadriceps Stretch:

Stand on one leg, holding onto a wall or chair for stability.

Bend your contrary knee, bringing your heel inside the route of your buttocks.

Hold your ankle and lightly pull your foot in the direction of your buttocks to stretch the the front of your thigh.

Hold for 20-30 seconds on each leg.

three. Wall Sits:

Stand together with your decrease again in competition to a wall.

Slide down the wall until your knees are bent at a 90-degree angle, as if you're sitting in a chair.

Hold this position for so long as you can, then pass back to a standing feature.

Chapter 5: Nutrition for Joint Health

Nourishing Your Joints: The Role of Nutrition in Joint Health

Our joints are super and tricky systems that permit us to transport, bend, and perform everyday sports activities. Whether you're an athlete aiming to beautify basic overall performance or a person searching out consolation from joint pain, the position of vitamins in joint health can't be underestimated. A balanced food plan wealthy in specific vitamins can manual the properly-being of your joints, lessen contamination, and promote usual joint flexibility and durability.

In this newsletter, we are capable of find out the importance of proper nutrients for joint health, spotlight key nutrients that play a essential characteristic, and offer sensible guidelines that will help you make knowledgeable nutritional picks that can benefit your joints for years yet to come. Whether you're a fitness fanatic, someone dealing with joint issues, or certainly trying to maintain joint health as you age, the records you advantage right here can empower you to take proactive steps within the route of a life with healthful, ache-free joints.

Foods That Promote Joint Health: Nourish Your Way to Pain-Free Living

Good joint health is critical for maintaining an energetic, ache-loose way of life. While exercising and way of life picks play a crucial feature, your weight loss program is similarly vital in phrases of supporting and promoting joint fitness. Certain meals are rich in vitamins that might assist reduce infection, protect cartilage, and enhance everyday joint function. In this article, we'll find out some of those joint-pleasant ingredients and why they need to be a normal a part of your diet.

1. Fatty Fish:

Fatty fish like salmon, mackerel, trout, and sardines are ok in omega-three fatty acids. These healthful fat have effective anti inflammatory houses that can help lessen joint ache and stiffness. Omega-3s additionally contribute to the general fitness of your joints with the useful resource of the use of promoting cartilage repair and protection.

2. Berries:

Berries, together with strawberries, blueberries, and raspberries, are complete of antioxidants, at the side of anthocyanins and eating regimen C. These antioxidants assist shield joint tissues from harm because of risky molecules referred to as free radicals. Regular consumption of berries can help mitigate infection and sluggish down the improvement of joint-associated situations.

three. Leafy Greens:

Leafy inexperienced greens like spinach, kale, and Swiss chard are rich in nutrients and minerals, which includes nutrients K and calcium. Vitamin K is critical for correct bone health, and strong bones are critical for supporting your joints. These veggies moreover encompass anti-inflammatory compounds which could make contributions to joint consolation.

4. Nuts and Seeds:

Nuts and seeds, together with almonds, walnuts, and flaxseeds, offer healthy fats, protein, and various vitamins and minerals. They are specially high in magnesium, which plays a function in muscle and nerve function. Maintaining sturdy and well-functioning muscle groups spherical your joints can help assist joint stability and reduce the danger of harm.

5. Turmeric:

Turmeric is a spice said for its effective anti inflammatory compound called curcumin. Regularly incorporating turmeric into your diet, each as a spice in cooking or within the shape of turmeric nutritional nutritional supplements, may additionally moreover additionally assist alleviate joint pain and reduce infection.

6. Garlic:

Garlic consists of sulfur compounds that have been associated with decreased symptoms of osteoarthritis. These compounds can also furthermore assist guard cartilage from harm and hold joint fitness over time.

7. Olive Oil:

Extra virgin olive oil is wealthy in monounsaturated fats and antioxidants, that have anti inflammatory residences. Using olive oil as your number one cooking oil can make contributions to a joint-satisfactory weight loss plan.

8. Bone Broth:

Bone broth is an superb source of collagen, a protein that makes up a massive part of cartilage and facilitates preserve joint integrity. Including home made or keep-

presented bone broth to your eating regimen can offer the building blocks your joints need.

A properly-balanced healthy dietweight-reduction plan that consists of those joint-high-quality meals can play a pivotal position in promoting joint health and dealing with joint-associated problems. Remember that vitamins is simply one piece of the puzzle; it have to be complemented via regular exercising, a healthful life-style, and proper clinic treatment if you have present joint situations. By making knowledgeable nutritional choices and nourishing your joints with the right factors, you could pave the way for a lifestyles with robust, bendy, and ache-unfastened joints.

Supplements and Their Role in Knee Health: Enhancing Joint Support

Knee health is a critical thing of not unusual mobility and nice of lifestyles, and it's no surprise that human beings are looking for diverse processes to beneficial resource and hold it. While a balanced food regimen and normal exercise shape the muse of knee fitness, dietary supplements may be treasured additions for your recurring. In this newsletter, we'll discover the position of nutritional dietary supplements in selling knee fitness, focusing on the ones who have proven promise in helping joint characteristic and reducing soreness.

1. Glucosamine and Chondroitin:

Glucosamine and chondroitin are of the maximum well-known dietary nutritional dietary supplements for joint fitness. They are herbal additives of cartilage, the tissue that cushions the ends of bones to your joints. Many people take the ones dietary supplements to ease joint ache and doubtlessly gradual the improvement of situations like osteoarthritis. While consequences range from person to individual, some studies suggest that glucosamine and chondroitin may also moreover moreover offer comfort for knee osteoarthritis signs and symptoms and signs and symptoms.

2. Omega-3 Fatty Acids:

Omega-three fatty acids, normally determined in fish oil nutritional dietary supplements, have powerful anti inflammatory houses. Chronic irritation is a key contributor to joint pain and harm. By reducing infection, omega-3s may additionally additionally help alleviate knee pain and beautify joint feature. It's essential to pick out splendid fish oil nutritional dietary supplements for max effectiveness.

three. Turmeric and Curcumin:

Turmeric, a famous spice, consists of curcumin, a compound with robust anti inflammatory and antioxidant homes. Curcumin dietary supplements have acquired interest for their capacity to reduce knee pain and enhance joint feature in humans with osteoarthritis. These supplements are frequently used as complementary treatments along different joint health measures.

4. Collagen Supplements:

Collagen is the principle structural protein in connective tissues, at the side of the ones placed inside the knee joint. Collagen dietary dietary supplements goal to assist joint fitness by presenting the body with the constructing blocks it needs to hold cartilage and joint integrity. While research is ongoing, some human beings document reduced joint ache and superior mobility with collagen supplementation.

Chapter 6: Pain Management Strategies

Pain Management Strategies for Healthy Knees

Knee pain is a commonplace sickness that might effect absolutely everyone, from athletes pushing their bodily limits to individuals navigating the worrying situations of growing vintage. Whether you're handling the ache of a current harm or dealing with continual knee ache, finding effective pain control techniques is essential to regain your mobility and outstanding of life.

In this complete manual, we're able to find out quite a few ache manage strategies in particular tailored to cope with knee ache. From manner of lifestyles adjustments to exercising workouts, nutritional picks, and present day treatment options, we'll provide you with the know-how and system you want to take control of your knee health. By the prevent of this guide, you'll be better prepared to make informed alternatives about a way to alleviate knee pain, improve joint feature, and embark on a journey to a ache-free, active life.

Coping with Knee Pain

Knee ache may be a day by day mission, impacting your mobility, independence, and preferred great of life. Whether it's due to damage, arthritis, or one of a kind situations, handling knee pain calls for a multifaceted approach that mixes clinical steering, lifestyle adjustments, and self-care techniques. In this newsletter, we'll explore effective approaches to control knee ache, so you can regain manage, reduce pain, and maintain residing life to the fullest.

1. Seek Medical Advice:

The first and maximum vital step in coping with knee ache is to trying to find recommendation from a healthcare expert. They can provide an accurate analysis, understand the underlying reason of your ache, and endorse suitable treatment alternatives. These may additionally

additionally encompass bodily treatment, treatment, injections, or maybe surgery if essential.

2. Maintain a Healthy Weight:

Excess weight places extra stress in your knees, exacerbating pain and pain. Losing weight through a balanced weight loss plan and regular exercising can substantially reduce the strain on your joints and assist alleviate knee pain.

3. Stay Active within Your Limits:

While it's crucial to stay active, it's similarly essential to pick out sports which is probably slight to your knees. Low-impact wearing events like swimming, biking, and water aerobics can assist preserve joint mobility and improve the encircling muscle groups without inflicting immoderate strain.

four. Physical Therapy:

Working with a bodily therapist may be immensely beneficial. They can broaden personalised exercising sporting activities to bolster your knees, beautify flexibility, and reduce pain. They may moreover use strategies like guide remedy and ultrasound to relieve pain.

5. Assistive Devices:

Using assistive gadgets like knee braces, canes, or crutches can assist reduce the pressure in your knees and offer more useful useful resource while wanted. These gadgets can make each day sports more viable and masses tons much less painful.

6. Pain Medication:

Over-the-counter ache relievers or prescription medicines advocated with the aid of your healthcare enterprise can assist manage knee ache. However, it's crucial to apply them as directed and be aware about functionality issue consequences.

7. Heat and Cold Therapy:

Applying warmness or bloodless packs to your knees can offer short remedy from ache and inflammation. Experiment with every techniques to appearance which one works terrific for you.

eight. Mind-Body Techniques:

Practices like meditation, deep respiration sports, and guided imagery let you control ache by way of promoting rest and lowering strain, that may exacerbate discomfort.

9. Dietary Choices:

Maintaining a balanced food plan wealthy in anti inflammatory food like fatty fish, culmination, vegetables, and entire grains can assist lessen contamination within the body, possibly assuaging knee ache.

10. Manage Stress:

Chronic ache often comes with emotional stress. Engage in strain-discount strategies like mindfulness, yoga, or counseling to enhance your intellectual and emotional nicely-being.

Coping with knee pain is a adventure that requires staying strength and staying power. By combining medical steering, life-style modifications, and self-care strategies, you can take big steps towards decreasing ache and improving your first-rate of life. Remember that during truth honestly all and sundry's enjoy with knee ache is unique, so it's essential to art work carefully together with your healthcare issuer to create a customized pain manipulate plan that incredible suits your needs.

Medication Options for Knee and Joint Pain

Knee and joint pain may be a continual and debilitating trouble, affecting loads of lots of humans worldwide. While there are various strategies to dealing with this discomfort, drug treatments are often a cross-to possibility for comfort. In this newsletter, we'll find out not unusual remedy alternatives for knee and joint ache, outlining their professionals and cons to help you make knowledgeable decisions approximately pain manage.

1. Nonsteroidal Anti-Inflammatory Drugs (NSAIDs):

Pros:

NSAIDs, to be had each over the counter (e.G., ibuprofen) and by the usage of the use of prescription (e.G., naproxen), are effective in lowering pain and infection.

They are widely available and can offer pretty fast consolation for slight to mild ache.

NSAIDs can enhance joint characteristic and mobility, making every day sports more feasible.

 Cons:

Long-time period or excessive use of NSAIDs can purpose gastrointestinal issues collectively with ulcers or bleeding.

Some humans might also additionally enjoy aspect consequences like stomach ache, heartburn, or kidney problems.

NSAIDs do not address the underlying reason of joint pain and might simplest provide temporary treatment.

2. Acetaminophen:

Pros:

Acetaminophen (e.G., Tylenol) is normally well-tolerated and masses less probably to reason gastrointestinal troubles in assessment to NSAIDs.

It can be effective for moderate to moderate ache comfort and is broadly available.

Cons:

Acetaminophen does no longer very own anti inflammatory residences and won't be as powerful for joint pain with giant contamination.

Excessive use can cause liver damage, making it critical to stick to encouraged dosage guidelines.

three. Opioids:

Pros:

Opioid drug treatments, like oxycodone and hydrocodone, are powerful pain relievers which can offer comfort for excessive joint pain.

They can be prescribed for brief-term use after surgery or for individuals with extreme pain that does not reply to exceptional remedies.

Cons:

Opioids bring a high threat of dependence, addiction, and overdose, making them wrong for lengthy-term ache manipulate.

Side outcomes can consist of drowsiness, constipation, and respiratory despair.

Long-term opioid use can motive tolerance, in which higher doses are required for the equal diploma of pain comfort.

four. Corticosteroids:

Pros:

Corticosteroid injections (e.G., cortisone) straight away into the joint can offer fast and focused consolation from infection and pain.

They are powerful for situations like osteoarthritis, rheumatoid arthritis, and bursitis.

Cons:

Repeated corticosteroid injections can weaken the encircling tissues and probably motive joint damage over time.

Short-time period aspect outcomes can also include transient pain or swelling at the injection net internet page.

five. Disease-Modifying Antirheumatic Drugs (DMARDs):

Pros:

DMARDs like methotrexate are used to deal with inflammatory joint situations like rheumatoid arthritis.

They can sluggish down the development of joint harm and enhance lengthy-term joint function.

Cons:

DMARDs may additionally take several weeks to months before their effects come to be big.

They might also have factor consequences, which incorporates liver and blood mobile abnormalities, requiring regular tracking.

Medications can be treasured machine in handling knee and joint ache, providing treatment and enhancing preferred great of life. However, it's crucial to weigh the experts and cons of every treatment possibility and communicate over with a healthcare business enterprise for custom designed steerage. Additionally, combining medicinal drug with one-of-a-kind strategies like bodily remedy, life-style modifications, and nutritional changes can provide a complete method to successfully managing knee and joint pain at the same time as minimizing capability dangers and detail consequences.

Alternative Pain Relief Methods for Joint Pain

Living with joint pain may be a every day struggle, impacting your mobility, comfort, and widespread pleasant of lifestyles. While medicines and bodily treatment are usually used to control joint ache, opportunity pain consolation strategies offer promising options that can supplement traditional remedies. In this article, we'll find out a number of those opportunity techniques, with a particular popularity on the capability blessings of cold-water immersion.

1. Physical Therapy and Exercise:

Physical treatment and centered exercising programs can assist enhance joint mobility, energy, and flexibility. A expert bodily therapist can layout customized workout workouts to cope with your precise joint issues, supporting to alleviate ache and beautify everyday joint characteristic.

2. Acupuncture:

Acupuncture, a conventional Chinese medicinal drug method, includes the insertion of skinny needles into particular elements on the body. Some humans record comfort from joint pain and advanced mobility following acupuncture instructions. While the mechanisms inside the lower returned of its effectiveness aren't simply understood, it's far considered a secure complementary remedy.

three. Heat and Cold Therapy:

Heat and cold therapy can offer temporary remedy from joint pain. Applying a warmth compress or taking a heat tub can assist loosen up muscle tissues and decrease stiffness, even as cold packs can help reduce contamination and numb pain.

four. Mind-Body Techniques:

Mindfulness meditation, relaxation bodily games, and guided imagery can assist manage the emotional and mental elements of ache. These practices can lessen strain and beautify your capability to cope with persistent joint pain.

5. Dietary Supplements:

Certain nutritional nutritional dietary supplements, which encompass glucosamine, chondroitin, and omega-3 fatty acids, are believed to aid joint fitness and decrease infection. Consult with a healthcare provider in advance than along side dietary dietary supplements for your routine to ensure protection and effectiveness.

6. Percussive Therapy:

In contemporary years, percussive remedy has obtained popularity as a flexible and effective technique to promoting popular properly-being. This modern method consists of using hand held devices that supply fast, targeted pulses or vibrations to the frame's gentle tissues. In this communicate, we're capable of discover the makes use of and benefits of percussive remedy, dropping mild on its developing role in enhancing bodily health and nicely-being.

1.   Muscle Recovery and Pain Relief: Percussive remedy is appreciably employed to relieve muscle pain, stiffness, and pain. Athletes, health fanatics, and those enhancing from accidents discover it particularly useful for enhancing muscle restoration and reducing publish-workout ache.

2.   Physical Performance Enhancement: Athletes and strolling footwear use percussive remedy as a part of their pre-exercise bodily sports. It lets in stimulate blood go with the float, beautify flexibility, and decorate muscle basic performance, getting prepared the frame for most fascinating average performance.

3.   Relief from Chronic Pain: Percussive treatment can offer comfort from continual situations in conjunction with fibromyalgia,

arthritis, and sciatica. Its deep tissue rubdown impact can help lessen pain and decorate ordinary comfort.

4.   Stress   Reduction: The   rhythmic percussive motions have a chilled effect at the frame, reducing pressure and selling rest. Many humans use it to unwind and de-pressure after an extended day.

Benefits of Percussive Therapy:

1.   Improved   Blood   Circulation: The speedy   pulses   of   percussive   treatment stimulate blood go with the flow to focused regions, facilitating the delivery of nutrients and oxygen to muscles and helping inside the removal of waste merchandise.

2.   Enhanced   Muscle   Recovery: By lowering muscle tension and pain, percussive remedy   accelerates   the   frame's   natural recuperation techniques, deliberating faster healing amongst physical games or injuries.

three. Increased Range of Motion: Regular use of percussive remedy can decorate joint flexibility and kind of motion. This is specifically beneficial for people with mobility problems.

four. Reduced Muscle Knots and Trigger Points: Percussive therapy enables break up muscle knots and trigger factors, which can be a full-size deliver of pain and decreased mobility.

five. Convenience and Accessibility: Handheld percussive devices make this remedy on hand to human beings inside the comfort of their homes. This consolation permits for additonal commonplace and ordinary use.

6. Non-Invasive: Percussive treatment is non-invasive and doesn't require the usage of medicines or invasive strategies, making it a stable and herbal approach to pain alleviation and fitness.

Percussive treatment has emerged as a powerful tool for promoting bodily fitness and general properly-being. Its programs variety from relieving muscle ache and dashing up recovery to improving athletic standard performance and decreasing pressure. As the recognition of percussive treatment keeps to boom, greater people are discovering the advantages of this innovative approach to properly-being. Whether you're an athlete on the lookout for to optimize popular performance, a person dealing with persistent pain, or sincerely searching out rest and strain comfort, percussive remedy gives a flexible and on hand solution that will help you gather your fitness desires.

7. Cold Water Immersion:

Cold water immersion, furthermore known as bloodless remedy or cryotherapy, is an possibility ache treatment method that has acquired interest for its capability benefits in dealing with joint pain. It includes immersing the affected region, which incorporates the knees or one of a kind joints, in bloodless water for a fantastic period.

Benefits of Cold-Water Immersion for Joint Pain:

Reduced Inflammation: Cold water can constrict blood vessels and reduce blood glide to the affected vicinity, which can also additionally help lessen contamination and alleviate ache.

Numbing Effect: The bloodless water can offer a numbing effect, short relieving pain by way of lowering the transmission of ache indicators to the brain.

Improved Joint Mobility: Some people discover that cold water immersion complements joint mobility, making it much less complicated to carry out physical video video games and sports activities.

How to Try Cold Water Immersion:

1.   Fill a tub with bloodless water (50-59°F or 10-15°C).

2.   Submerge the affected joint or frame element for about 10-15 minutes, or till it becomes uncomfortably cold.

3.   Repeat this technique as wanted, permitting the pores and skin to transport decrease lower back to its regular temperature among schooling.

8. Intra-Articular Injections for Knee Pain:

We will find out what intra-articular injections are, how they artwork, and their capability advantages in assuaging knee pain.

Understanding Intra-Articular Injections:

Intra-articular injections are a kind of remedy wherein remedy is introduced without delay into the joint region of the knee. This method permits for centered remedy, addressing pain and infection on the supply. The maximum used drugs for intra-articular injections encompass corticosteroids and hyaluronic acid.

How Intra-Articular Injections Work:

1.   Corticosteroids: These   anti inflammatory   medicinal   capsules   can unexpectedly lessen infection and pain inside the   knee   joint.   They   art   work   through suppressing   the   immune   response   that triggers   inflammation.   Corticosteroid injections can offer exceedingly short remedy, regularly interior a few days to each week.

2.   Hyaluronic Acid: Also referred to as Visco   supplementation,   hyaluronic   acid injections   goal   to   restore   the   natural lubrication and cushioning within the knee joint. This can assist reduce friction and ease pain   associated   with   situations   like osteoarthritis. The effects of hyaluronic acid injections may additionally additionally take some weeks to end up important and can ultimate for numerous months.

Chapter 7: Adaptive Equipment and Gear

Living with knee pain or constrained knee mobility may be hard, however it doesn't need to mean giving up your active manner of life or independence. Adaptive equipment and equipment specifically designed to assist and accommodate lousy knees might also need to make a significant distinction for your every day life. In this introductory article, we can discover the area of adaptive device and tool tailor-made to people with knee troubles, highlighting how the ones innovative gear can empower you to hold mobility and regain control over your sports.

From assistive devices like knee braces and canes to adaptive apparel and mobility aids, the alternatives to be had are various and cater to severa goals. Whether you're getting better from surgical treatment, handling chronic knee pain, or absolutely looking for techniques to make each day life more snug, you'll find out that adaptive device and tools can play a pivotal position in improving your common well-being.

In the articles to study, we will delve deeper into unique kinds of adaptive device and tools, offering insights into their functions, advantages, and the way they may be integrated into your daily recurring. Whether you're searching out solutions to resource your independence at home, decorate your mobility outside, or honestly beautify your first-rate of existence with awful knees, the world of adaptive device and tool has a few factor to provide all people. So, permit's embark on a journey to find out the equipment and improvements that will let you stay your life to the fullest, irrespective of your knee-related traumatic situations.

The Importance of Proper Footwear

When it includes coping with knee issues and maintaining joint fitness, we often cognizance on carrying events, treatments, and medications. However, one essential detail is regularly neglected – right shoes. The footwear you select out to position on can extensively effect your knee health and not unusual properly-being. In this text, we'll find out the importance of right shoes for knee issues and why selecting the proper footwear is a crucial step in managing knee-related demanding situations.

1. Shock Absorption:

The knees bear a massive amount of effect with every step you are taking. Proper footwear with accurate enough marvel absorption can assist cushion those affects, lowering the pressure to your knee joints. Shoes with cushioned insoles and supportive midsoles are first rate alternatives for humans with knee troubles.

2. Stability and Support:

Shoes with fantastic arch aid and right balance abilties can assist preserve accurate alignment and reduce the chance of overpronation or supination, that would stress the knees. Look for footwear that offer desirable enough ankle beneficial resource as well, as ankle stability is intently associated with knee fitness.

3. Reduced Pain and Discomfort:

Ill-turning into or unsupportive shoes can exacerbate knee pain and ache. Shoes that provide a cushty but snug healthy can assist distribute your body weight more lightly and alleviate stress at the knees. This can be especially useful for people with situations like osteoarthritis or tendonitis.

4. Enhancing Mobility:

The right footwear can decorate your commonplace mobility and make it a whole lot less tough to have interaction in physical sports sports and sports that sell knee health. Properly equipped shoes can enhance your self assure in shifting around, likely encouraging you to stay active and hold joint flexibility.

5. Injury Prevention:

Wearing footwear perfect for your particular desires and sports can lessen the hazard of knee accidents. For instance, if you're a runner, choosing taking walks shoes that provide the proper aid and cushioning can assist prevent overuse accidents that regularly have an impact at the knees.

6. Custom Orthotics:

For individuals with particular knee troubles or irregularities in foot shape, custom orthotic inserts prescribed via a podiatrist or orthopedic professional can be lifestyles converting. These inserts are designed to provide customized manual and alignment tailor-made to your precise goals.

Proper shoes is a critical difficulty of knee health that must no longer be underestimated. The proper shoes can provide critical marvel absorption, balance, and assist, helping to reduce ache, ache, and the chance of harm. When dealing with knee problems, it's encouraged to speak over with a podiatrist or orthopedic expert who can test your individual needs and recommend suitable footwear or custom orthotics. By taking the time to pick out the proper footwear in your knee fitness, you're taking a proactive step in the route of enhancing your famous well-being and ensuring a more comfortable and energetic life.

Mobility Aids and Devices for Bad Knees

Living with horrible knees can notably impact your mobility, making even smooth duties hard. However, the world of mobility aids and devices gives numerous contemporary answers that will help you regain your independence and beautify your excellent of lifestyles. In this article, we'll discover severa mobility aids and devices designed specifically for humans with knee problems, highlighting how they are able to empower you to transport with self guarantee and ease.

1. Canes:

Canes are a number of the maximum common mobility aids and are available in severa patterns, which includes unmarried-point canes, quad canes, and forearm crutches. They offer stability and aid at the identical time as walking, decreasing the pressure on your knees, and supporting to keep stability.

2. Knee Scooters:

Knee scooters are an high-quality opportunity to standard crutches. These devices permit you to rest your injured knee on a cushioned platform with wheels, allowing you to move spherical with out bearing weight on the affected knee. They are particularly useful for humans recuperating from knee surgical methods or accidents.

three. Walkers:

Walkers offer great balance and useful resource, making them ideal for people with excessive knee issues. They frequently include add-ons like trays and baskets for added consolation all through each day sports activities.

four. Orthopedic Knee Braces:

Orthopedic knee braces provide centered aid and compression to the knee joint. They can assist stabilize the knee, lessen ache, and enhance mobility. Different varieties of knee braces are available, consisting of those designed for particular situations like osteoarthritis or ligament injuries.

5. Mobility Scooters:

For people with extra considerable mobility demanding situations, mobility scooters provide a cushty and handy way to get spherical. These electric powered scooters are suitable for both indoor and out of doors use, presenting a greater diploma of independence.

6. Elevating Leg Rests:

Elevating leg rests are often implemented in aggregate with wheelchairs or mobility scooters. They will will will let you decorate and useful aid the affected leg, lowering swelling and pain inside the knee joint.

7. Stairlifts and Ramps:

For people with knee troubles that have an effect on their capability to navigate stairs, stairlifts and ramps can be worthwhile. They ensure steady and smooth get entry to to special levels of your private home.

8. Adaptive Clothing:

Adaptive garb is designed with abilties like Velcro closures, smooth-get right of entry to zippers, and adjustable closures to simplify the method of having dressed, especially for humans with constrained knee mobility.

Mobility aids and gadgets play a critical feature in enhancing the independence and excellent of lifestyles for humans with awful knees. These equipment offer help, reduce pain, and make it much less complex to carry out every day activities and preserve an active way of life. When considering mobility aids, it's crucial to talk over with a healthcare expert or bodily therapist to decide the most suitable options on your unique desires. By embracing those devices, you can regain your mobility and preserve to live lifestyles to the fullest, irrespective of your knee-related worrying situations.

Home Modifications for Accessibility

For human beings with awful knees, the residence can once in a while experience like an impediment direction complete of demanding situations. However, with thoughtful domestic adjustments, you can create a greater available and snug living surroundings that enables your mobility and independence. In this text, we'll discover diverse domestic adjustments tailored to individuals with knee troubles, imparting realistic solutions to make each day lifestyles extra feasible.

1. Handrails and Grab Bars:

Installing handrails and draw close bars in key areas of your home, together with the relaxation room, staircases, and hallways, can offer thousands-desired assist and balance.

These smooth additions can assist in standing up, sitting down, and navigating your private home safely.

2. Non-Slip Flooring:

Replacing slippery floors with non-slip alternatives can help prevent accidental falls. Consider textured tiles or non-slip mats in areas just like the relaxation room and kitchen, wherein water and spills are common.

3. Ramp Installation:

For homes with steps major to the doorway, putting in ramps can make sure easy get admission to for human beings with constrained knee mobility or those the usage of mobility aids. Portable ramps also are to be had for transient use.

4. Widening Doorways:

Widening doorways can accommodate mobility aids like wheelchairs or walkers and offer extra region to transport with no trouble, specially if you have to navigate slim hallways or tight corners.

5. Lever-Style Door Handles:

Replace traditional doorknobs with lever-fashion handles which can be less complicated to apprehend and carry out, requiring an lousy lot less dexterity and strain.

6. Raised Toilet Seats:

A raised rest room seat can make it a good deal much less complicated to sit down down down and get up from the relaxation room, decreasing strain at the knees. Some fashions furthermore encompass armrests for introduced manual.

7. Shower Bench or Chair:

A bathe bench or chair allows you to sit whilst showering, lowering the want to stand for extended intervals, which can be difficult for lousy knees. Pair it with a handheld showerhead for added comfort.

Chapter 8: Finding Community Support and Community

Embarking on a journey to keep an energetic and healthful way of life with lousy knees can sometimes revel in like a solitary corporation. However, there's a wealth of resource and community assets to be had to help you in this direction. In this introductory article, we'll discover the importance of looking for manual and connecting with local sources, businesses, and prefer-minded people who percent your willpower to overcoming knee-related worrying situations.

1. Support Groups:

Support organizations, whether in-individual or on line, provide a precious platform for people with awful knees to attach, percentage opinions, and exchange advice. These groups provide emotional assist and practical insights, helping you navigate the physical and emotional elements of knee-related situations.

2. Physical Therapy and Rehabilitation Centers:

Physical remedy facilities aren't only locations for professional guidance but additionally hubs of network resource. These centers frequently host employer remedy classes and workout instructions tailored to human beings with knee issues, fostering a feel of camaraderie amongst contributors.

3. Fitness and Wellness Clubs:

Many fitness and wellness clubs provide specialized applications and commands designed for human beings with limited knee mobility. These commands popularity on low-effect carrying activities and are led with the beneficial resource of instructors experienced in running with people with knee issues.

4. Local Parks and Recreation Departments:

Local parks and exercising departments frequently put together outdoor sports activities appropriate for all health degrees. Whether it's moderate taking walks groups, outdoor yoga commands, or senior fitness packages, the ones sources assist you to live energetic on the identical time as gambling the splendor of the outdoor.

five. Healthcare Providers and Physical Therapists:

Your healthcare issuer or physical therapist can characteristic a treasured resource for statistics approximately close by resource groups and assets. They also can offer steerage on wearing activities, remedy alternatives, and manner of life adjustments to higher manage knee-associated conditions.

6. Online Communities:

The digital age has introduced about an abundance of on line communities, forums, and social media groups wherein people with similar challenges be a part of and percentage advice. These virtual areas can be specially beneficial for finding beneficial useful resource and property from the comfort of your private home.

Seeking aid and community assets is a important step in your journey to last lively and healthy with lousy knees. These networks provide encouragement, data, and motivation, making it a lot much less tough to overcome boundaries and live dedicated for your properly-being goals. Whether you're seeking out emotional guide, exercise partners, or steering on navigating every day lifestyles with knee issues, there's a network equipped to welcome you. So, take that first step, hook up with others, and discover the wealth of assets to be had to help you lead a fulfilling and energetic life, irrespective of your knee-related challenges.

Joining Local Senior Fitness Groups

Aging gracefully and maintaining an energetic manner of existence are dreams shared by using many seniors, and close by senior fitness companies can be instrumental in reaching those goals. These companies provide a supportive, attractive surroundings wherein humans can stay healthy, socialize, and enhance their often going on nicely-being. Surprisingly, a few seniors even venture into CrossFit, a immoderate-intensity fitness recurring frequently associated with extra younger athletes. In this article, we'll find out the advantages of turning into a member of network senior fitness groups, together with the possibility of collaborating in CrossFit, and the way they might make contributions for your vibrant, healthy manner of life.

1. Community and Camaraderie:

One of the most good sized benefits of joining neighborhood senior fitness corporations is the feel of network they provide. These agencies offer a threat to satisfy like-minded people who percent your passion for staying energetic and wholesome. The friendships forged right right here may be a supply of motivation and help as you pursue your health dreams.

2. Tailored Workouts:

Senior health agencies usually provide workouts and workout exercises tailored to the best desires and abilties of older adults. These carrying activities cognizance on improving flexibility, balance, strength, and cardiovascular health, all of which can be critical for fashionable health and harm prevention.

three. Social Interaction:

Participating in company health sports can combat feelings of isolation and loneliness, which may be common amongst seniors. Regular social interaction has been proven to have numerous highbrow and emotional advantages, contributing to a excessive first-class outlook on life.

4. CrossFit for Seniors:

CrossFit, stated for its intensity and practical movements, might probably appear intimidating at the start, but it's an increasing number of attracting seniors seeking out a project. Some CrossFit gyms provide changed exercising routines particularly designed for older adults, emphasizing proper shape, protection, and gradual development. These modified CrossFit commands can help seniors decorate electricity, agility, and endurance at the same time as pushing their barriers in a supportive surroundings.

five. Improved Physical Health:

Regular bodily interest, whether or not or not thru senior fitness groups or CrossFit, can motive severa health blessings, which includes stepped forward cardiovascular fitness, stronger muscle power, better bone density, and progressed flexibility. These benefits contribute to greater independence and durability.

6. Cognitive Health:

Physical exercise has a outstanding effect on cognitive function and may help reduce the risk of cognitive decline. Engaging in business enterprise health sports disturbing conditions the mind and frame, stimulating highbrow agility and reminiscence.

7. Sense of Achievement:

Achieving health milestones, whether or not it's mastering a brand new yoga pose or finishing a hard CrossFit workout, can beautify conceitedness and provide a experience of fulfillment. These victories may be specifically profitable for seniors searching for to keep an lively way of life.

Joining close by senior health businesses, which includes the possibility of exploring changed CrossFit applications, is a fantastic way for older adults to stay active, related, and engaged in lifestyles. These groups provide tailored exercising routines, a experience of network, and numerous physical and highbrow health blessings. Whether you're searching for to preserve your fitness, make new buddies, or mission yourself in new techniques, senior fitness agencies provide a supportive environment wherein you can hold to thrive as you age gracefully.

Virtual Support Networks and Resources

In in recent times's virtual age, finding beneficial aid and resources for staying lively with horrific knees has in no manner been less complicated, way to the energy of virtual organizations and on line systems. Whether you're seeking out steerage, motivation, or a enjoy of reference to like-minded humans, digital guide networks offer a wealth of opportunities to help you overcome knee-associated disturbing conditions and preserve an energetic way of life. In this article, we'll discover the advantages of tapping into those online sources and the way they're capable of make contributions on your journey toward higher knee fitness and standard nicely-being.

1. Online Forums and Communities:

Online forums and groups committed to knee fitness and fitness provide a vicinity wherein human beings can percentage their studies, ask questions, and provide assist and recommendation. These systems be a part of you with people who understand the worrying situations of awful knees and can provide valuable insights and encouragement.

2. Virtual Exercise Classes:

Numerous fitness studios and instructors now provide virtual exercise schooling that cater to people with knee troubles. Whether it's low-effect yoga, seated aerobics, or focused energy training, the ones schooling permit you to participate from the comfort of your house even as receiving professional steering.

3. Social Media Support Groups:

Social media systems like Facebook and Instagram host groups and pages devoted to knee health and lively developing older. Joining these organizations may be a part of you with a broader community of oldsters which might be obsessed on keeping an lively way of life regardless of knee annoying situations.

four. Telehealth Consultations:

Telehealth services will allow you to go to healthcare companies, bodily therapists, and health experts from the ease of your private home. They can take a look at your situation, provide custom designed workout workout routines, and provide steerage on coping with knee-associated issues.

five. YouTube Tutorials:

YouTube is a treasure trove of health and rehabilitation tutorials. Many bodily therapists and health professionals percent academic motion pix on knee-particular sports activities sports, stretches, and strategies to enhance mobility and decrease pain.

6. Mobile Apps:

There are numerous mobile apps designed to help human beings with knee troubles music their improvement, set dreams, and get proper of access to exercise workouts. These apps often include interactive skills and reminders to maintain you on course.

7. Online Challenges and Accountability Groups:

Participating in online fitness demanding conditions or becoming a member of obligation businesses can offer motivation and shape on your fitness habitual. These organizations often foster a experience of camaraderie and friendly competition, encouraging you to stay committed in your dreams.

Virtual useful useful resource networks and sources have transformed the manner individuals with awful knees can get right of access to facts, motivation, and steering to maintain an energetic manner of lifestyles. By connecting with the ones on-line organizations and using virtual structures, you may get right of access to a wealth of expertise and useful useful resource tailored on your specific desires. Whether you're seeking out exercise workouts, recommendation on managing knee pain, or surely a experience of belonging indoors a network of like-minded humans, those digital resources are treasured belongings on your adventure to higher knee fitness and sizeable nicely-being.

Success Stories and Inspiration

Aging gracefully and staying lively are goals loved with the useful resource of many seniors, even though faced with the mission of lousy knees. The testimonies of these who've triumphed over adversity, defying the restrictions of knee problems, function effective assets of proposal for others. In this newsletter, we'll discover fulfillment reminiscences and percentage inspirational stories of seniors who have not high-quality embraced an active lifestyle however have thrived however their knee-related demanding situations.

1. The Power of Determination:

Meet John, a retiree who grow to be an avid hiker earlier than his knee problems commenced. Diagnosed with intense osteoarthritis, he faced the possibility of a sedentary lifestyles. Undeterred, John sought the steerage of a professional physical therapist who helped him boom a custom designed exercising plan targeted on low-impact sports sports like swimming and table positive cycling. Over time, his strength of mind and endurance paid off, and he not excellent regained his ability to hike however additionally climbed his first mountain positioned up-analysis. John's story underscores the importance of strength of will and professional steering in overcoming knee stressful situations.

2. Yoga for Resilience:

Mary, a retired schoolteacher, faced debilitating knee pain because of years of harm and tear and tear. Fearful of surgery, she have become to yoga for a extra holistic technique to her restoration. With the steerage of a certified yoga trainer skilled in running with seniors and knee problems, Mary started out a slight yoga workout. Through constant strive and endurance, she frequently advanced her flexibility and knee power. Mary's story highlights the capacity of yoga as a recovery tool for seniors with awful knees.

three. Adaptive Sports Triumph:

Sam, a former athlete, confronted the disappointment of a knee damage that brought on chronic ache. Instead of giving in to depression, Sam explored adaptive sports activities for individuals with disabilities. He found wheelchair basketball, a tough and dynamic game that not best furnished an exceptional workout but additionally a newfound experience of cause. Sam's journey reminds us that possibilities for staying lively can be located in surprising places, despite the fact that faced with huge knee issues.

4. The Joy of Community:

Sarah, a retiree residing in a senior network, located out the importance of companionship in her quest to stay active with terrible knees. She initiated a strolling business enterprise internal her network, bringing together fellow citizens who shared her motive. With the resource of her newfound friends, Sarah located motivation to walk regularly, even on days at the same time as her knees protested. Her tale emphasizes the function of community and social assist in preserving an active manner of lifestyles.

Chapter 9: Sustaining Your Active Lifestyle

Maintaining an active life-style is a cornerstone of a wholesome and gratifying existence, but for those managing terrible knees, the route to staying active can now and again seem uncertain and difficult. The desirable information is that horrible knees need now not be a roadblock in your nicely-being. In this comprehensive manual, we're capable of discover strategies, guidelines, and insights with a purpose to empower you to preserve your active manner of lifestyles even as coping with knee issues effectively.

Our adventure will take us thru the worlds of adaptive device, low-impact bodily video video games, energy and versatility education, nutrients for joint health, pain management, and loads greater. Whether you're a senior in search of to live active, an athlete getting better from knee accidents, or someone handling persistent knee issues, this manual is designed to provide you with the records and gear to thrive regardless of the boundaries.

As we delve into the various elements of maintaining an active manner of lifestyles with terrible knees, recollect that your adventure is precise, and there may be nobody-duration-suits-all method. Instead, we'll equip you with a toolkit of strategies and options, allowing you to tailor your approach in your unique needs and dreams. With strength of will, expert guidance, and a immoderate exceptional thoughts-set, you can navigate the worrying conditions of terrible knees and maintain to guide a colourful, lively existence that complements your regular nicely-being. So, permit's embark in this adventure together, as we find out the strategies to keep your active way of life and thrive within the face of knee-associated demanding conditions.

Crafting a Sustainable Fitness Plan

As we age, staying bodily active turns into an increasing number of essential for our ordinary health and well-being. For seniors handling the task of terrible knees, it's important to create a long-term health plan that no longer best allows a healthful lifestyle however additionally addresses precise knee-related troubles.

Maintaining an active and healthy manner of life is essential for seniors, irrespective of age or physical traumatic conditions like terrible knees. Crafting a protracted-term health plan tailored in your man or woman desires will will assist you to live energetic, improve your ordinary properly-being, and manage knee-associated problems effectively. In this brief article, we'll outline the crucial element steps to help seniors craft a sustainable fitness plan that promotes mobility, energy, and preferred health, all at the equal time as looking after their knees.

1. Consult with a Healthcare Professional:

Before embarking on any health journey, it's vital to speak over along side your healthcare issuer or orthopedic expert. They can have a look at your precise knee troubles, offer guidance on exercise suitability, and offer tips tailored for your scenario.

2. Set Clear and Realistic Goals:

Define your fitness desires, whether or not or now not or no longer it's improving knee flexibility, increasing electricity, or improving preferred mobility. Setting smooth and manageable desires will preserve you inspired and provide a sense of motive to your fitness recurring.

3. Prioritize Low-Impact Activities:

For seniors with terrible knees, low-effect sports sports are frequently the safest and first-rate desire. Activities like swimming, water aerobics, desk bound biking, and gentle yoga vicinity minimal pressure at the knee joints whilst supplying outstanding cardiovascular blessings and muscle strengthening.

4. Embrace Strength and Flexibility Training:

Incorporate strength and versatility sporting sports activities into your health plan. Focus on strengthening the muscle businesses around the knee joint, as this could provide introduced useful resource and decrease knee pain. Resistance bands, body weight physical video games, and changed weightlifting wearing events are remarkable options.

five. Start Slow and Progress Gradually:

Begin your fitness journey with mild, low-depth sports and step by step growth the depth, duration, and complexity through the years. Avoid the temptation to push too hard too rapid! Gradual development is crucial to fending off harm and constructing sustainable fitness. Start with plausible physical video video games and often boom intensity, length, and complexity as your energy and mobility enhance.

6. Listen to Your Body:

Always be aware about how your frame feels for the duration of and after workout. If you enjoy pain or soreness beyond mild muscle ache, it's important to regulate or save you the exercise. Your safety and well-being need to continually come first.

7. Balance Cardiovascular and Strength Training:

A properly-rounded fitness plan want to encompass each cardiovascular and strength schooling elements. Cardiovascular sports activities activities beautify coronary coronary coronary heart fitness, at the same time as power training preserves muscular tissues and joint feature.

eight. Stay Consistent:

Consistency is essential to long-time period fulfillment. Create a normal exercising time desk that you may realistically keep on with. Consistency permits gather behavior and guarantees you continue to acquire the blessings of physical interest.

nine. Warm-Up and Cool Down:

Never pass your warmth-up and funky-down sports. These segments prepare your body for exercising, reduce the threat of harm, and promote flexibility and healing.

10. Seek Professional Guidance:

Consider running with an authorized personal trainer or physical therapist skilled in working with seniors and knee problems. Their know-how will will let you design a customized and solid fitness plan.

Creating an extended-time period fitness plan for seniors with awful knees is an funding to your fitness and properly-being. By consulting with healthcare professionals, setting possible goals, prioritizing low-effect sports activities sports, and embracing electricity and versatility education, you may craft a sustainable health recurring that lets in you to guide an active and pleasurable existence regardless of knee-associated disturbing conditions. Remember, the essential component to achievement is sluggish development, consistency, and taking note of your frame, ensuring that your health adventure is each secure and interesting.

Creating a protracted-term fitness plan for seniors with horrible knees is a proactive step closer to maintaining a wholesome and active lifestyle. By looking for expert advice, setting conceivable dreams, incorporating low-impact sports, and prioritizing strength and flexibility education, seniors can craft a fitness ordinary that now not high-quality addresses knee-associated stressful conditions but also complements common well-being. Remember, sluggish development, consistency, and taking note of your frame are the keys to a a success and sustainable health adventure that allows every your knee fitness and your commonplace energy.

Monitoring Progress and Adjusting

Staying energetic after 60 with lousy knees isn't always pretty a good deal beginning a health habitual; it's about retaining one which adapts for your converting wishes and progresses step by step. Monitoring your development and making essential changes alongside the manner are important to make sure you can maintain taking detail inside the blessings of an active way of existence on the same time as safeguarding your knee fitness. In this short article, we'll discover the importance of monitoring your health adventure and a manner to make knowledgeable changes for extended-term fulfillment.

1. Keep a Fitness Journal:

Start via preserving a fitness magazine. Record your exercising workouts, which incorporates the sports activities, period, and intensity. Note any adjustments on your knee ache, mobility, or conventional properly-being. A magazine gives a easy picture of your development through the years.

2. Set Milestones and Goals:

Establish unique milestones and desires to your fitness journey. These can encompass growing the duration of your walks, improving your form of motion, or accomplishing extra power in your leg muscle tissues. Having clean objectives offers you some component to artwork in the course of.

3. Regularly Assess Your Knee Health:

Schedule ordinary checks together with your healthcare enterprise or bodily therapist to evaluate america of the united states of your knees. They can provide insights into any modifications to your condition and provide guidelines to regulate your health plan because of this.

four. Listen to Your Body:

Pay close to interest for your frame's signs all through and after workout. If you revel in expanded ache, discomfort, or swelling in your knees, it's crucial to take it significantly. These signs may also propose the need for adjustments for your habitual.

five. Adapt and Modify Exercises:

As you improvement, it's essential to comply and modify your sporting sports to undertaking yourself at the equal time as shielding your knees. Consult with a health professional to research new sports or techniques that align at the side of your desires and limitations.

6. Explore Different Modalities:

Consider incorporating different forms of sports activities into your routine. For instance, if on foot will become difficult, try swimming or water aerobics. Variety no longer only maintains your recurring engaging however additionally dreams outstanding muscle organizations.

7. Seek Professional Guidance:

Consult with a llcensed personal teacher or bodily therapist who focuses on jogging with seniors and knee issues. They can examine your improvement, alter your exercising workout routines, and offer ongoing steerage to make certain your regular stays effective and safe.

eight. Be Patient and Persistent:

Progress might not continually be linear, and there may be setbacks along the way. It's crucial to stay affected person and continual, know-how that retaining an energetic way of life is a long-time period dedication.

9. Stay Informed:

Keep updated with the present day research and trends related to knee health and fitness for seniors. New techniques, physical sports activities, and strategies can also moreover emerge that might benefit your habitual.

10. Embrace a Holistic Approach:

Remember that staying energetic is in reality one part of a holistic approach to well-being. Proper vitamins, proper enough relaxation, and strain manipulate additionally play crucial roles in maintaining common fitness.

Monitoring your progress and making knowledgeable changes are critical factors of staying active after 60 with awful knees. By preserving a health mag, putting dreams, regularly assessing your knee health, and searching out expert guidance, you may make sure that your fitness ordinary evolves to assist your changing wishes and maintains to beautify your normal super of existence. Adapting to new challenges and persevering through setbacks will allow you to enjoy the blessings of an lively manner of existence well into your senior years at the equal time as searching after your knee health.

Celebrating Achievements and Embracing the Future

The journey of staying lively after 60 with lousy knees is complete of triumphs, big and small, that deserve birthday celebration. As you navigate the stressful situations, modify, and persist for your efforts, it's essential to pause and acknowledge your achievements alongside the manner. In this brief article, we'll discover the importance of celebrating the ones milestones and the manner to set your attractions on the thrilling opportunities that lie in advance.

1. Reflect on Your Journey:

Take a 2nd to reflect on how a long way you've come because of the reality you released into your fitness journey. Think approximately the enhancements on your knee health, mobility, and commonplace properly-being. Whether it's on foot longer distances, studying new bodily games, or experiencing reduced pain, every fulfillment is a testomony on your determination and resilience.

2. Acknowledge Small Wins:

Don't underestimate the significance of small victories. Every step you're taking toward better knee health, and an active way of life is certainly well worth celebrating. It may be as smooth as finishing a hard exercise or constantly sticking on your exercising routine.

3. Set New Goals:

As you have fun your achievements, look in advance, and set new desires on your fitness adventure. These desires can be both health-related and private, together with completing a 5K walk, attempting a brand new low-impact exercise beauty, or maybe exploring a particular shape of health altogether. Having new dreams maintains your motivation immoderate.

4. Embrace New Adventures:

Staying active after 60 can be a gateway to new adventures and opinions. Whether it's joining a hiking group, taking part in a network event, or visiting to find out new landscapes, an energetic life-style opens doorways to interesting possibilities.

5. Continue Learning:

Stay curious and maintain gaining knowledge of about health, vitamins, and knee health. The greater you realize, the higher prepared you are to make knowledgeable selections and modify your health plan as favored.

6. Share Your Success:

Share your achievements with friends and family. Not best will this provide you with a feel of pride, however it is able to additionally encourage and inspire others to embark on their very own health trips.

7. Embrace a Positive Mindset:

Maintain a powerful mind-set as you have got an first-rate time your achievements and appearance in advance. Cultivate optimism and resilience, know-how that stressful situations are a herbal part of the journey, and your self-discipline will see you thru.

Chapter 10: Knee Arthritis

Knee arthritis is an infection that impacts the knee joint and consequences in swelling, ache, and stiffness. The thigh bone (femur), shin bone (tibia), and kneecap make up the knee joint (patella). The cartilage that connects the ones bones serves as a cushion in most of the bones. This cartilage starts offevolved to come to be worse in people with knee arthritis, allowing the bones to rub within the path of each other and ensuing in swelling and pain.

There are severa types of knee arthritis, with osteoarthritis and rheumatoid arthritis being the maximum trendy.

The maximum ordinary kind of knee arthritis is known as osteoarthritis, and it's miles added on by the usage of the cartilage within the knee joint progressively deteriorating through the years. The time period "placed on-and-tear" arthritis is often used to give an reason for this shape of arthritis, this is extra common in older individuals.

An inflammatory condition called rheumatoid arthritis outcomes in contamination of the joints, specifically the knee joint. This kind of arthritis may moreover have an effect on numerous joints at some diploma within the frame and is extra ordinary in younger persons.

People may want to in all likelihood have particular knee arthritis signs and symptoms, however common ones embody:

Pain, specially at the equal time as on foot or fame

stiffness, specially within the morning or after spending hundreds of time sitting

Knee joint swelling and inflammation

decreased knee kind of movement

People with more immoderate knee arthritis may additionally moreover need to discover it hard to stroll, stand, or climb stairs.

Knee arthritis may be crippling and substantially lessen someone's extremely good of existence. Reduced signs and symptoms and symptoms and slowed illness development are made feasible by early evaluation and treatment.

Prevalence of Knee Arthritis in Older Adults

Among aged folks, knee arthritis is a wellknown illness. Over 50% of human beings over the age of sixty 5 are idea to have some shape of knee arthritis for the cause that incidence of the situation rises with age. As a end result, one of the maximum conventional causes of impairment in older men and women is knee arthritis. It affects extra ladies than person adult males.

Risk Factors for Knee Arthritis in Older Adults

Numerous factors might also make it more likely for older oldsters to growth knee arthritis. These include:

Age: As formerly said, as people age, their chance of growing knee arthritis rises.

Obesity: Increased put on and strain on the knee joints may furthermore cease end result from being obese or obese.

Previously injured knee: The chance of acquiring knee arthritis after a previous harm is advanced.

Genetics: Some people may additionally additionally moreover have a hereditary susceptibility to knee arthritis.

Occupation: Certain jobs that require a number of heavy lifting or repeated kneeling may growth your danger of growing knee arthritis.

Knee arthritis can also be made more likely with the aid of using wonderful clinical problems together with diabetes, high blood pressure, and coronary heart illness.

It's essential to remember that no matter the reality that these threat elements could probably enhance your danger of getting knee arthritis, they do not always cause it. Older humans may additionally additionally take movement to save you or take away the improvement of knee arthritis with the aid of being aware of the ones risk factors.

KNEE ARTHRITIS SYMPTOMS AND DIAGNOSIS

Common Symptoms of Knee Arthritis

People may have special knee arthritis symptoms and signs, however frequent ones encompass:

Pain: Knee arthritis regularly manifests as ache, which may be something from a touch ache to a strong, excruciating suffering. When fame or shifting approximately, pain is often extra, and resting or slumbering down may additionally additionally make it go away.

Stiffness: Another desired sign of knee arthritis is stiffness. This may be greater apparent in the morning or after prolonged intervals of sitting.

Swelling and infection: Knee arthritis signs which includes swelling and infection within the knee joint may be present. To the contact, the knee may also additionally experience heated.

Reduced form of motion: As arthritis worsens, the knee can also stiffen and end up extra difficult for the person to move. This also can make it tough to stand, walk, or climb stairs.

Cracking or popping sounds: When they float their knee joint, a few sufferers may additionally additionally moreover concentrate or experience cracking or popping noises.

Grinding sensation: Some people may additionally moreover have a grinding feeling interior their knee.

It's important to keep in mind that the ones signs and signs and signs also can be brought on via other ailments, so it is constantly higher to get a prognosis from a physician. To verify the analysis, a healthcare practitioner is probably capable of behavior a bodily exam, compare a affected individual's scientific data, and possibly request imaging tests like x-rays or MRI.

The maximum everyday signs of knee arthritis are the ones already indexed, although some human beings may have uncommon symptoms. Some human beings must have knee ache or stiffness that continues them up at night time, at the same time as others would possibly limp, enjoy wiped out, or battle with smooth everyday obligations like dressing or taking walks. Some sufferers additionally may be feverish, which might be a signal of a joint contamination. It's vital to get clinical help in case you or a person is affected by any of these symptoms and signs and symptoms and signs and symptoms.

Diagnostic Tests and Imaging for Knee Arthritis

Physical exam, collectively with a check of the affected individual's medical history, are commonly the primary steps in the analysis of knee arthritis. A scientific practitioner will check the knee joint for symptoms of stiffness, ache, and contamination. They might also inquire about any signs and symptoms or signs and symptoms and signs, which includes soreness or problem strolling, in addition to any beyond ailments or traumas to the knee that might have prompted the onset of arthritis.

Diagnostic tests and imaging may be requested to verify the presence of knee arthritis and take a look at the situation's severity. These embody:

X-rays: can be used to see the knee's bones and joints and to locate any changes, which includes bone spurs or cartilage deterioration.

MRI (Magnetic Resonance Imaging): MRI is a non-invasive imaging approach that produces satisfactory-grained pictures of the knee joint the usage of a magnetic discipline and radio waves. It is probably useful to appearance how the knee's ligaments, clean tissues, and cartilage are doing.

CT (Computerized Tomography) take a look at: A CT take a look at is each different imaging check which could offer precise pix of the knee joint. It additionally can be used to show the abilities of the bones and to devise operations.

Ultrasound: An ultrasonic imaging technique that employs sound waves to offer images of the knee joint is non-invasive. It might be useful to look how the knee's ligaments, smooth tissues, and cartilage are doing.

Blood checking out: Blood assessments may be required to rule out specific ailments that may resemble knee arthritis signs and symptoms, collectively with rheumatoid arthritis, gout, or lupus.

The sort of knee arthritis and the severity of the sickness can be recognized the usage of those diagnostic strategies, which will assist decide the extremely good direction of treatment.

A healthcare practitioner may make use of numerous diagnostic equipment to evaluate the knee joint and its characteristic similarly to the diagnostic exams and imaging indicated above. These embody:

Joint aspiration: A needle is brought into the joint in the course of a joint aspiration operation to retrieve a touch amount of fluid for trying out. You may also additionally take a look at the fluid for symptoms of infection or contamination.

Knee arthroscopy: During a surgical procedure known as knee arthroscopy, a tiny virtual virtual camera is used to have a take a look at the knee joint inner. It can be used to find out any underlying sicknesses that might be inflicting knee pain, in addition to to diagnose and cope with knee arthritis.

Gait assessment is the act of reading someone's on foot sample to pick out any irregularities or asymmetries inside the knee joint's motion.

Muscle and energy finding out: This examination will observe the electricity of the quadriceps, hamstrings, and calf muscle organizations, which manual the knee.

All of those imaging studies and diagnostic system can also aid clinical practitioners in successfully diagnosing knee arthritis and deciding on the affected character's fine path of treatment.

Differentiating among Osteoarthritis and Rheumatoid Arthritis

The maximum frequently taking place styles of knee arthritis are osteoarthritis and rheumatoid arthritis, but every has particular origins, signs and symptoms, and remedies.

Osteoarthritis is a degenerative illness that develops through the years whilst the cartilage within the knee joint little by little wears away. It is introduced on with the resource of things like age, obesity, and in advance knee injuries. Pain, stiffness, and a discounted style of motion within the knee are a number of its signs. The bone may additionally moreover boom spur-like projections and the joint may also expand. Osteoarthritis, every so often known as "located on-and-tear" arthritis, is more huge in older people.

An inflammatory situation referred to as rheumatoid arthritis results in contamination of the joints, in particular the knee joint. The lining of the joint is attacked via using the immune tool in this shape of arthritis, causing infection and destruction. It is characterized by the usage of signs and symptoms and signs such as knee joint pain, stiffness, and oedema. Additionally, it is able to have an impact on many joints inside the direction of the frame, and more youthful women and men are more susceptible to it.

The healthcare organisation may additionally additionally utilize the diagnostic techniques and imaging techniques already mentioned, as well as blood checks to look for nice markers, such as rheumatoid factor, which can be often located in rheumatoid arthritis.

It's important to bear in mind that there are numerous functionality reasons for knee arthritis, making it vital to talk with a healthcare issuer for a specific analysis and the fine direction of movement.

Chapter 11: Treatment Options for Knee Arthritis

Knee Arthritis Medications and Dietary Supplements

To manipulate the signs and signs and symptoms and signs and symptoms of knee arthritis and lessen joint irritation, many drugs and dietary supplements may be employed. Among the most usually used prescribed drugs and nutritional nutritional nutritional dietary supplements are:

NSAIDs (non-steroidal anti inflammatory pills): These drugs, in conjunction with ibuprofen and naproxen, also can furthermore useful resource in reducing discomfort and infection inside the knee joint.

Acetaminophen: is a painkiller that might useful resource in easing discomfort and ache in the knee joint.

Corticosteroids: Prednisone is one example of a corticosteroid that may be used to lessen infection inside the knee joint. They may be injected really into the joint or taken with the aid of way of mouth.

Disease-enhancing anti-rheumatic pills (DMARDs): These drug remedies, together with methotrexate, can be used to gradual the development of rheumatoid arthritis and reduce contamination in the joint.

Biologic response modifiers (biologics): These tablets, which consist of adalimumab, may be used to lessen knee joint infection and decrease the advancement of rheumatoid arthritis.

Glucosamine and chondroitin: This complement might also furthermore assist to delay the direction of osteoarthritis and beneficial resource to relieve pain and contamination inside the knee joint.

Before beginning any new treatment, it is vital to undergo in mind the feasible risks and advantages with a healthcare expert and hold in mind that some pills and nutritional supplements might also additionally have adverse results. The perfect route of remedy for an man or woman may also need some trial and errors for the reason that numerous drugs and supplements may work in every other manner for splendid people. Along with one-of-a-kind non-medicinal alternatives like bodily remedy and workout, a healthcare expert may go with you to growth an effective remedy plan that includes treatment and dietary supplements to control the signs and symptoms of knee arthritis.

Physical Therapy and Exercise for Knee Arthritis

Exercise and bodily treatment are critical elements of the treatment of knee arthritis. They may additionally moreover resource in easing ache, enhancing mobility, and delaying the deterioration of the sickness.

Physical remedy: Physical treatment may moreover help to lessen discomfort, improving the form of motion, and strengthening and flexing the knee joint. Exercises that concentrate on the knee joint and the muscle agencies that assist it may observe via the use of a bodily therapist. To reduce the strain at the knee joint, they may additionally teach the affected man or woman how to utilize aids like canes, walkers, or crutches.

Exercise: Regular exercise can also moreover help to growth flexibility, relieve pain, and give a boost to the muscle mass that assist the knee joint. Additionally, exercise may additionally help to lower the hazard of falling and enhance desired fitness. For human beings with knee arthritis, low-impact sports like swimming, cycling, and water aerobics are suitable choices. The energy of the knee joint may also be accelerated with the aid of doing strengthening sports activities sports which incorporates leg presses, calf lifts, and knee extensions.

When beginning an exercise software for knee arthritis, it is critical to have interaction with a scientific expert or physical therapist. They might also moreover assist in developing a customized exercising software program that takes the individual's requirements and dreams into interest, further to evaluates improvement and make changes as critical.

It's essential to recall that bodily remedy and exercising need to be accomplished below the supervision of a systematic practitioner and which you need to constantly be aware of your frame.

If you experience pain or discomfort whilst exercising, it's miles essential to prevent or regulate your exercising and are searching for clinical advice. Additionally, it's miles crucial, first of all, low-intensity exercising exercises and frequently boom every duration and depth over the years. To study development and advantages over time, it's also important to stick to the exercise schedule constantly.

Other non-scientific measures, along side coping with weight, the use of assistive era, and making modifications to the living environment, may assist to reduce pressure at the knee joint and increase mobility further to exercise and bodily remedy.

It's important to hold in mind that there can be no treatment for knee arthritis; however, with the proper care, inclusive of drugs, nutrients, bodily treatment, workout, and manner of life modifications, human beings with knee arthritis may additionally moreover moreover manipulate their signs and symptoms and symptoms and signs and symptoms and beautify their exceptional of life.

Physical remedy wearing activities and sports activities for human beings with arthritis inside the knee are to be had in loads of bureaucracy. Several times encompass:

Range of motion physical video games: Exercises that boom variety of motion are alleged to increase the knee joint's flexibility and mobility. Exercises for the knees in flexion and extension, ankle pumps, and calf stretches are a few examples.

Strengthening physical video games: Exercises that enhance muscular power and help the knee joint are referred to as strengthening sporting activities. Leg presses, calf lifts, and knee extensions are a few examples.

Aerobic bodily activities: Aerobic Exercises can also additionally assist to increase cardiovascular fitness, reduce pain, and decorate fashionable fitness. Examples of cardio sports activities encompass walking, swimming, biking, and water aerobics.

Exercises for balance: By improving stability and balance, the ones physical sports may also moreover additionally lower the threat of falling and increase mobility. Tai chi, a unmarried-legged posture, and heel-toe taking walks are the severa examples.

Exercises for joint safety: These actions are imagined to lessen the stress on the knee joint and enhance common joint fitness. As an instance, consider taking brief breaks at the same time as popularity or sitting for prolonged durations, in addition to working within the direction of right object movement and lifting strategies.

Stretching bodily sports activities: Exercises that expand the muscle tissue may additionally moreover additionally loosen them up and increase flexibility. Stretches for the quadriceps, hamstrings, and calves are some examples.

It's crucial to make bigger a specialized exercising software program with the assist of a bodily therapist or any other healthcare professional that takes into attention the character's requirements, goals, and present diploma of fitness. It's crucial to pay attention in your body and chorus from physical games that make you sense ache or pain. You need to additionally begin with low-depth bodily sports and gradually increase the depth and period through the years.

Additionally, counting on the type and diploma of knee arthritis, a few humans may additionally moreover gain extra from effective sports. People with superior osteoarthritis, for example, would in all likelihood benefit greater from sports that target joint safety and type of motion, even as humans with early-stage osteoarthritis should possibly gain more from bodily games that focus on strengthening and growing muscle useful useful resource throughout the knee joint.

Additionally, it is critical to keep in mind that physical treatment and sports need to be completed beneath the supervision of a healthcare professional. A healthcare professional want to moreover be consulted in advance than beginning any new exercise software. Maintaining a everyday exercise agenda is likewise important if you want to look improvements and advantages through the years.

It's important to engage with a healthcare practitioner to increase a selected remedy plan that takes into hobby the individual's requirements and dreams to manipulate the signs and symptoms of knee arthritis and decorate mobility.

Surgery and different invasive techniques

In splendid situations, treating knee arthritis may furthermore encompass surgical treatment or fantastic invasive remedies. These remedies may additionally moreover reduce ache, boom mobility, and hold all over again the situation's improvement. Surgery and other invasive remedies have to great be used as a final resort while all one-of-a-type healing options have failed.

Examples of invasive and surgical remedies for knee arthritis include:

Knee joint alternative: The injured knee joint is changed with an synthetic joint at some point of a surgical operation known as a knee opportunity. Depending at the diploma of the injury, both a complete or partial knee substitute can be used to perform this.

Knee arthroscopy: A tiny digital camera is used throughout a surgical procedure called a knee arthroscopy to test the knee joint from the internal. It can be used to find out any underlying ailments that is probably inflicting knee soreness, similarly to to diagnose and deal with knee arthritis.

Osteotomy: This surgical treatment, it truely is greater normal in the early stages of osteoarthritis, involves reducing and reshaping the bone to reduce strain on the joint.

Cartilage restore: Repairing or changing the broken cartilage within the knee joint is the surgical manner known as cartilage repair.

Synovial fluid alternative: A needle is introduced into the joint to extract a tiny amount of fluid for evaluation and alternative with synthetic or donated synovial fluid in the course of the synovial fluid replacement operation.

It's crucial to remember that those operations consist of sizable dangers and results and want healing time. Before opting to have surgery or any invasive treatment, it's miles important to keep in mind the possible risks and advantages with a healthcare practitioner.

Surgery is regularly most effective determined on as a final inn or whilst different remedies have failed or the damage is excessive. The first line of treatment normally consists of bodily remedy, workout, medicinal drug, and weight manipulate.

LIFESTYLE AND DIET CHANGES FOR MANAGING KNEE ARTHRITIS

The significance of maintaining a healthful weight

For people with knee arthritis, keeping a wholesome weight is critical thinking about that it may assist to increase mobility and reduce strain on the knee joint. As more weight locations more pressure at the knee joint, which also can motive contamination, soreness, and stiffness, weight issues is a massive hazard aspect for developing knee arthritis.

In addition to worsening the symptoms of knee arthritis, being obese increases the risk of obtaining additional diseases together with diabetes, coronary coronary heart illness, and excessive blood pressure.

Both the threat of getting knee arthritis and the signs and signs of knee arthritis can be controlled by means of the usage of losing weight. Losing even a hint amount of weight also can have a big impact on enhancing mobility and reducing knee joint pressure.

It's vital to consume a balanced weight loss plan this is high in cease result, greens, complete grains, and lean protein while proscribing processed food, sugar, and saturated fat to hold a healthy weight. Regular exercise can also moreover assist you burn strength and hold a wholesome weight, which includes taking walks, swimming, biking, and water aerobics.

It's critical to take into account that weight reduction want to be completed healthily and sustainably, with the assist of a healthcare expert. It's additionally crucial to be aware of your frame and live some distance from excessive or restrictive diets.

In prevent, ladies and men with knee arthritis should try and hold a healthy weight on account that doing so may additionally assist to growth mobility, reduce strain on the knee joint, and beneficial useful resource to keep away from extraordinary health issues.

Exercise and physical interest pointers for seniors with Knee Arthritis

The benefits of bodily hobby and exercise for elderly humans with knee arthritis include ache relief, improved mobility, and a slowed charge of sickness development. It's crucial to don't forget that seniors may additionally have distinct bodily restrictions and can want to adjust their exercise ordinary.

For seniors with knee arthritis, the subsequent recommendations for workout and bodily hobby:

Low-impact sports activities sports: Walking, swimming, cycling, and water aerobics are some examples. These ache-free exercising workouts can also help to growth cardiovascular health, reduce soreness, and decorate massive health.

Exercises for constructing power: Knee extensions, leg presses, and calf lifts are a few examples. These sports activities sports also can useful useful useful resource in strengthening the muscles that manual the knee joint.

Range-of-movement bodily sports: Exercises that decorate style of motion consist of calf stretches, ankle pumps, and knee flexion and extension physical sports. These physical video games may additionally aid in enhancing the knee joint's flexibility and mobility.

Balance sporting activities: Examples of stability physical sports include heel-toe walking, tai chi, and single-leg stances. These carrying activities also can moreover aid in growing stability and balance, which can lessen the risk of falling and growth mobility.

Stretching wearing occasions: Hamstring, quadriceps, and calf stretches are some examples. These wearing activities can also ease irritating muscle companies and boom flexibility.

In addition to starting with low-intensity sporting occasions and step by step growing the depth and length over the years, it's far essential to collaborate with a bodily therapist or some distinct healthcare expert to develop a custom designed exercising plan that takes into consideration the character's needs, dreams, and modern degree of fitness. It's critical to pay attention to your frame and steer easy of any sports that make you feel pain or ache.

Seniors ought to frequently workout and be physical lively, but it is also essential to get medical recommendation earlier than beginning any new health recurring and to be aware of the frame's signs, taking breaks when critical.

When it entails exercising and physical hobby, seniors with knee arthritis have additional elements to don't forget.

Gradual improvement: It's vital to start gently and building up your exercising program's duration and depth frequently over the years.

Listen for your frame: Seniors want to be aware of their our our bodies and refrain from painful or uncomfortable exercising exercises. They must additionally prevent within the occasion that they enjoy any pain or ache while workout.

Use assistive devices: To reduce stress on the knee joint, seniors also can benefit from the use of assistive system like canes, walkers, or crutches.

Monitoring: Seniors should regularly examine their symptoms and signs and improvement, and change their workout ordinary as essential.

Combine workout with particular treatments: For the nice results, exercise have to be used alongside aspect different treatment plans which consist of treatment, bodily remedy, and weight manipulate.

Safety: Seniors need to keep away from workout workouts which may be too difficult or that positioned them in risk of falling. Safety is a few detail that should be taken significantly.

It's additionally critical to don't forget that physical interest and workout ought to be accomplished underneath the supervision of a healthcare practitioner and which you have to talk with a healthcare expert earlier than beginning any new exercise routine. Seniors with knee arthritis need to have interaction in everyday workout because it enables ease signs and symptoms and symptoms, increase mobility, and halt the ailment's development.

Diet and Nutrition for Knee Arthritis Management

Diet and nutrients can play an critical feature in handling the signs of knee arthritis. A healthful food regimen can assist to reduce infection, enhance commonplace fitness, and sell weight reduction. Here are some dietary and nutritional hints for human beings with knee arthritis:

Anti-inflammatory foods: Include meals which might be excessive in anti inflammatory compounds, at the side of omega-3 fatty acids (positioned in fatty fish which incorporates salmon and sardines), antioxidants (determined in give up end result and vegetables), and flavonoids (found in berries, cherries, and citrus fruits).

Fibre-wealthy meals: Include components which may be immoderate in fibre, which incorporates culmination, vegetables, whole grains, and legumes. Fibre permits to reduce contamination and promote weight loss.

Lean protein: Include lean protein property which includes fish, hen, turkey, tofu, and legumes. Protein is important for constructing and repairing muscle groups.

Limit processed ingredients: sugar and saturated fat can increase infection and make contributions to weight gain.

Supplements: Some dietary nutritional supplements, which include glucosamine and chondroitin, also can assist to reduce ache and contamination in the knee joint and might gradual the development of osteoarthritis. However, it is vital to talk about using nutritional supplements with a healthcare expert in advance than beginning any new supplement everyday.

Hydration: Adequate hydration is essential for everyday fitness and the lubrication of joints.

It's essential to study that everybody's nutritional desires are one-of-a-kind, and it's miles vital to are looking for for advice from a healthcare expert or a

a registered dietitian to create a custom designed dietary plan that takes into attention the character's desires and goals.

It's moreover critical to recall that nutritional modifications should be made step by step and in a sustainable way, and need to be combined with ordinary workout and physical interest, further to other treatments which encompass medicine and physical treatment, for exceptional consequences.

It's important to make certain that the diet regime affords all the critical nutrient the frame need which incorporates vitamins, minerals and macronutrients, and to ensure the weight loss program is balanced and consistent with the man or woman's nutritional hints and goals.

In precis, a healthful weight loss plan and vitamins can play an essential characteristic in dealing with the symptoms and signs of knee arthritis via lowering inflammation, selling weight loss, and improving wellknown fitness. It's crucial to paintings with a healthcare professional or a registered dietitian to create a personalized nutritional plan that takes into account the character's goals and dreams.

FOOD TO AVOID

Certain substances may additionally exacerbate contamination and need to be restricted or prevented inside the healthy dietweight-reduction plan of people with knee arthritis. These encompass:

Fried elements: Fried food are immoderate in saturated and trans fat, that can boom infection.

Processed food: Processed food are often immoderate in sugar, salt, and artificial additives, that may growth irritation and make contributions to weight advantage.

Red meat: Red meat is immoderate in saturated fat, that could growth contamination.

Refined carbohydrates: Refined carbohydrates which encompass white bread, pasta, and sugar can purpose weight benefit and boom contamination.

Alcohol: Consuming immoderate alcohol can increase infection and exacerbate knee pain.

Nightshade veggies: Nightshade greens along side tomatoes, peppers, eggplants, and white potatoes have been stated to annoy infection in some human beings.

Chapter 12: Pain Management and Improving Mobility

Strategies for Managing Pain

Living with knee arthritis consists of gaining knowledge of to control your pain. There are numerous strategies for controlling pain, together with:

Medication: Acetaminophen and nonsteroidal anti-inflammatory drug treatments (NSAIDs), which may be to be had over-the-counter, may be used to deal with ache. Prescription pills like opioids and corticosteroids can be administered in extra intense circumstances. To find out the wonderful route of motion for a person's necessities, it's miles critical to talk about medicine usage with a healthcare practitioner.

Physical remedy and exercise: Exercise and physical remedy might also assist to increase mobility, lessen ache, and prevent the deterioration of the ailment. Exercises that target the knee joint and the muscle groups that assist it can benefit facts of thru a bodily therapist.

Weight control: Retaining a healthful weight may also additionally assist to decorate mobility and reduce stress at the knee joint.

Heat and cold remedy: Applying warmth or bloodless to the affected joint can assist to reduce ache and stiffness.

Acupuncture: Traditional Chinese clinical method referred to as acupuncture includes setting tiny needles into sure frame web sites. It is perception to resource in lowering infection and pain.

Massage: Massages also can ease pressure and pain in the muscle tissues, boom flow into, and activate relaxation.

Mind-body practices: Mind-frame practices like yoga, tai chi, and meditation can also assist reduce pain and anxiety, and enhance relaxation.

To pick out the extremely good route of motion for a person's requirements, it is vital to speak with a healthcare practitioner. Additionally, it's miles critical to maintain in thoughts that ache control is a persistent way, and if the soreness keeps, you ought to speak with a healthcare company.

It's moreover essential to keep in thoughts that once the illness worsens and the man or woman's dreams vary through the years, pain manage techniques might also moreover moreover want to be changed. It's vital to collaborate with a healthcare practitioner to create an extensive ache control method that mixes loads of strategies.

Other strategies for coping with ache encompass:

Assistive machine: Assistive device, which include canes, walkers, and crutches, can useful aid to beautify mobility and reduce stress on the knee joint.

Occupational remedy: Using strategies that placed tons a great deal much less stress on the knee joint, occupational remedy can also help humans with knee arthritis discover ways to perform normal responsibilities.

Transcutaneous Electrical Nerve Stimulation (TENS): TENS is a non-invasive method that makes use of electric powered impulses to reduce ache and infection.

Bracing: Wearing a knee brace can also assist to reduce the soreness thru helping and stabilizing the knee joint.

Lifestyle modifications: Lifestyle adjustments may additionally help to reduce pain and beautify elegant fitness. Examples encompass minimizing stress, getting genuine sufficient sleep, and giving up smoking.

It's vital to maintain in mind that handling pain is a chronic technique, and it's far essential to speak with a healthcare agency if the pain keeps or worsens. There are numerous processes to govern ache, so it's far essential to collaborate with a healthcare expert to create an all-encompassing ache manipulate technique that consists of some of techniques.

Techniques for reinforcing mobility and lowering stiffness

For elders with knee arthritis, developing mobility and reducing stiffness are crucial targets. To accomplish those goals, an entire lot of techniques can be carried out, which consist of:

Physical treatment and exercise: By strengthening the muscles that assist the knee joint and increasing the sort of movement, bodily remedy and exercising can also assist to increase mobility and reduce stiffness. Exercises that target the knee joint and the muscle groups that assist it can be trained with the aid of a physical therapist.

Therapy with warm temperature or bloodless may likely help to relieve pain and stiffness in the joint.

Massage treatment: Massage remedy allows ease tension inside the muscular tissues, increase blood drift, and encourage rest.

Assistive device: Assistive device, which encompass canes, walkers, and crutches, can beneficial resource to enhance mobility and lessen pressure at the knee joint.

Occupational remedy: Using techniques that located lots a good deal less pressure on the knee joint, occupational treatment may additionally help seniors who've knee arthritis.

Bracing: Wearing a knee brace also can additionally assist to stabilize and assist the knee joint, which allows reduce ache and stiffness.

Lifestyle adjustments might also help to lessen ache and beautify preferred health. Examples encompass minimizing stress, getting perfect sufficient sleep, and giving up smoking.

Other moderate sporting events collectively with yoga, tai chi, and others can also useful resource in enhancing mobility and lowering stiffness.

In addition, it's far important initially low-depth wearing activities and regularly increase the intensity and duration over the years. This should be completed at the side of a healthcare professional, which embody a physical therapist or a consultant in geriatric care, to create a customized plan that takes beneath interest the person's wishes, goals, and current level of fitness.

Assistive Devices and Equipment

Seniors with knee arthritis may moreover furthermore gain notably from the use of assistive equipment and device to increase mobility and decrease the pressure at the knee joint. The following are a few times of assistive system and device:

Canes: Canes can also help to lessen pain and increase mobility by means of helping and stabilizing the knee joint.

Walkers: Walkers provide the knee joint more stability and assist, which might also additionally lessen pain and increase mobility. Seniors also can moreover circulate approximately extra without trouble considering that there's a basket to hold their belongings.

Crutches: Crutches provide the knee joint extra stability and assist, which also can assist to lessen soreness and boom mobility. Seniors who aren't capable of go through weight on the injured knee might also moreover advantage the most from them.

Knee brace: A knee brace also can additionally assist to relieve soreness and boom mobility thru supporting and stabilizing the knee joint.

Elevated relaxation room seat: By minimizing the angle at which a senior with knee arthritis want to bend their knee, an extended lavatory seat might probably make using the relaxation room a lot less tough for them.

Shower chair: By removing the want to face at the identical time as getting showered, a bath chair can also make it a lot less complicated for seniors with knee arthritis.

Handrails: When ascending stairs or moving into and far from mattress, handrails also can provide help and stability.

Reacher: Seniors with knee arthritis may moreover furthermore use a reacher to choose up gadgets without bending over.

When strolling is uncomfortable and hard, an electric powered powered scooter or wheelchair can be carried out as a form of mobility help.

Other aids and furnishings are available that might be beneficial for aged human beings who've arthritis of their knees. Here are some one-of-a-type times:

Ramps: Ramps may also make trekking stairs and navigating choppy terrain less complicated for aged humans with knee arthritis.

Grab bars: In the toilet and other rooms of the house, grab bars may additionally moreover furthermore offer balance and help.

Adaptive utensils: By disposing of the need to hold or bend the fingers, adaptive utensils may also additionally make eating much less complex for seniors with knee arthritis.

Certain cushions: When seated, unique cushions might also additionally boom knee joint comfort and manual.

Slip-on shoe: Slip-on footwear may additionally additionally make placing on and starting off shoes for elderly people with knee arthritis less tough.

Stair carry: By doing away with the want to ascend the steps, a stair carry can also additionally make it less complicated for seniors with knee arthritis to manoeuvre them.

When motion is notably confined, seniors with knee arthritis may also employ a strength wheelchair due to the reality that they might perform it with a joystick and bypass at a quick tempo.

It's important to keep in thoughts that assistive devices and device need to be selected depending at the necessities and abilities of the person. To discover the proper gadgets and machine for a person's needs, it is essential to talk with a healthcare issuer or an occupational therapist.

Chapter 13: Improving Quality Of Life

Coping with the emotional and psychological factors of knee arthritis

The emotional and highbrow fitness of seniors may be significantly suffering from knee arthritis. Frustration, sadness, and despair may additionally give up stop end result from the scenario's pain, stiffness, and restricted movement. The following are a few coping mechanisms for dealing with the mental and emotional consequences of knee arthritis:

Acceptance: Seniors may additionally discover calm and control by the use of the usage of accepting the scenario and studying to stay with it.

Support: Seniors may moreover explicit their mind and gain useful resource from others who're going through similar conditions through turning into a member of a guide group or talking to a counselor.

Positive questioning: Thinking surely might also moreover help to lessen feelings of frustration and depression through way of encouraging humans to pay attention on what they're able to do in preference to on what they can't.

Maintaining social connections: Keeping up with buddies and circle of relatives may also offer you emotional guide and a revel in of direction.

Planning and placing practical dreams: Planning and growing sensible goals may also moreover additionally deliver seniors a experience of success and purpose them to experience greater on pinnacle of factors of their daily sports.

Maintaining interest and engagement: Maintaining hobby and engagement in pursuits, interests, and unique hobbies can also offer elders a revel in of path and assist a superb perspective.

Relaxation strategies: Deep breathing, yoga, and meditation are all powerful rest techniques that might help you enjoy better emotionally and reduce pressure.

Everyone has unique emotional and mental necessities, consequently it's miles vital to maintain in thoughts this and are searching out the advice of a counselor or a healthcare enterprise to pick out out the best course of movement.

Other techniques for coping with the mental and emotional results of knee arthritis encompass:

Keeping a magazine: Keeping a diary may additionally assist elders technique their emotions and beautify information in their scenario. Writing down mind, feelings, and evaluations can useful useful resource seniors.

Seeking expert counseling: A intellectual fitness expert may also provide assist, path, and coping mechanisms for managing the emotional and mental outcomes of knee arthritis. Seeking expert remedy.

Exercise: Regular exercising also can assist seniors preserve a sense of independence and self-reliance, that may beautify conceitedness and reduce depressive signs and symptoms and signs and symptoms.

Finding one-of-a-kind techniques of doing sports would probable help older humans hold their independence and feeling of control.

Keeping a sense of humor: Laughter may help seniors deal with the highbrow and emotional consequences of knee arthritis.

Practicing mindfulness: By challenge mindfulness bodily video video games, elders might also additionally learn how to give attention to the proper right here and now in area of focusing at the past or stressful about the future.

It's crucial to maintain in mind that the highbrow and emotional outcomes of knee arthritis can also modify through the years. If you continue to revel in signs and symptoms of melancholy or anxiety, you have got to speak with a psychologist or a healthcare agency. It's crucial to preserve a nice outlook and to invite for help from circle of relatives and buddies.

Support corporations and belongings

Seniors with knee arthritis may additionally find a whole lot of gain from help networks and splendid services. Seniors have the risk to percentage their reviews, studies from others, and get help from individuals who are aware of their struggles. For seniors with knee arthritis, the subsequent are some examples of help agencies and assets:

The Arthritis Foundation: is a national organization that gives beneficial resource, assets, and records to humans with arthritis. They provide some of services and sports activities, which includes instructional instructions, health applications, and aid groups.

Chapter 14: Present Research and Advice

Updates at the most modern-day findings about knee arthritis

New discoveries and enhancements are typically being made within the location of knee arthritis studies; this is dynamic and persevering with. Here are a few updates on contemporary knee arthritis research:

Biologic drugs: Biologic medicinal drugs: Biologic capsules inclusive of TNF inhibitors and interleukin-1 inhibitors have grow to be increasingly more well-known for treating knee arthritis. These medicinal tablets intention precise inflammatory pathways inside the body and were validated to be powerful in lowering ache and infection.

Stem mobile remedy: Stem cellular remedy is a notably new remedy opportunity for knee arthritis that includes injecting stem cells into the affected joint. Research suggests that stem cell remedy may be effective in decreasing pain and improving characteristic in human beings with knee arthritis.

Platelet-wealthy plasma therapy: Platelet-rich plasma remedy (PRP) is a treatment choice for knee arthritis that involves injecting a focused solution of platelets into the affected joint. Research indicates that PRP can be effective in decreasing ache and enhancing characteristic in human beings with knee arthritis.

Hyaluronic acid injections: Hyaluronic acid is a substance that is obviously gift within the body and is used to lubricate and cushion joints. Research indicates that hyaluronic acid injections may be effective in reducing ache and improving feature in people with knee arthritis.

Weight manage: Research shows that preserving a healthy weight can assist to lessen strain on the knee joint and enhance effects in human beings with knee arthritis.

Exercise: Studies have shown that workout is robust in reducing ache, enhancing characteristic, and slowing the improvement of knee arthritis. Exercise which incorporates cycling, swimming and water aerobics are mainly useful as they placed an awful lot a good deal much less strain on the knee joint.

It's critical to phrase that studies on knee arthritis is ongoing and new findings may additionally emerge. It's crucial to visit a healthcare professional to determine the maximum appropriate treatment for an character's goals.

Future remedies and upgrades

Future treatments and upgrades for senior with knee arthritis are being researched and advanced constantly. Here are some examples of destiny remedies and improvements that may be available for seniors with knee arthritis within the destiny:

Gene remedy: Gene therapy is a treatment that targets to intention the underlying causes of knee arthritis by way of introducing new genes or editing contemporary genes. This stays within the early degrees of studies however it is believed that it is able to be a promising treatment desire within the future.

Tissue engineering: Tissue engineering is a place of research that targets to create new tissue, which include cartilage, to replace damaged tissue in the knee joint. This remains in the early degrees of research but it's far believed that it is able to be a promising treatment opportunity in the destiny.

Robotics-assisted surgical remedy: Robotics-assisted surgical treatment is a way that makes use of a robotic arm to perform surgical operation with greater precision and accuracy. This technology is already being used for knee alternative surgical remedy and researchers are walking on developing robots that can perform extra complicated surgical techniques for knee arthritis.

Virtual reality treatment: Virtual truth therapy is a generation that allows sufferers to revel in a digital environment that simulates real-existence scenarios. This era is already being used for bodily remedy and researchers are running on developing digital truth environments that can be used for knee arthritis patients.

Artificial intelligence (AI): AI is being increasingly used in the scientific challenge to assist inside the analysis and remedy of various diseases. Researchers are working on growing AI-powered systems that may assist physicians in the analysis of knee arthritis and inside the improvement of custom designed treatment plans.

It's crucial to notice that those treatments are even though within the early tiers of studies and improvement, and it can be several years earlier than they'll be widely available. It's vital to talk over with a healthcare expert to decide the maximum appropriate remedy options to be had within the intervening time.

Monitoring: Seniors want to regularly determine their symptoms and improvement, and trade their workout routine as vital.

Combine exercise with unique remedy plans: For the fine consequences, workout want for use alongside element precise remedy plans which encompass remedy, bodily therapy, and weight manage.

Safety: Seniors need to keep away from carrying events which can be too difficult or that placed them in hazard of falling. Safety is a few thing that must be taken considerably.

It's moreover critical to maintain in mind that bodily activity and exercise need to be completed underneath the supervision of a healthcare practitioner and that you have to speak with a healthcare professional in advance than starting any new workout everyday. Seniors with knee arthritis have to engage in normal exercising since it permits ease symptoms and signs, growth mobility, and halt the disease's development.

Diet and Nutrition for Knee Arthritis Management

Diet and vitamins can play an essential feature in coping with the symptoms of knee arthritis. A healthy food regimen can help to lessen infection, improve everyday health, and sell weight loss. Here are some nutritional and dietary tips for people with knee arthritis:

Anti-inflammatory meals: Include foods which can be excessive in anti-inflammatory compounds, collectively with omega-3 fatty acids (placed in fatty fish which incorporates salmon and sardines), antioxidants (positioned in stop give up result and greens), and flavonoids (determined in berries, cherries, and citrus end end result).

Fibre-rich foods: Include meals which might be immoderate in fibre, which incorporates fruits, greens, complete grains, and legumes. Fibre allows to lessen inflammation and sell weight loss.

Lean protein: Include lean protein resources together with fish, chicken, turkey, tofu, and legumes. Protein is crucial for constructing and repairing muscle businesses.

Limit processed factors: sugar and saturated fats can growth infection and make a contribution to weight gain.

Supplements: Some dietary dietary supplements, together with glucosamine and chondroitin, can also assist to lessen pain and contamination in the knee joint and can sluggish the improvement of osteoarthritis. However, it's miles important to talk about using nutritional nutritional supplements with a healthcare professional earlier than starting any new supplement routine.

Hydration: Adequate hydration is crucial for preferred fitness and the lubrication of joints.

It's essential to be aware that everyone's nutritional dreams are terrific, and it's miles crucial to are looking for recommendation from a healthcare professional or a

www.ingramcontent.com/pod-product-compliance
Lightning Source LLC
Chambersburg PA
CBHW051727020426
42333CB00014B/1184